CW00677184

The Bariatric Blueprint

A Simple Guide to a Successful Lifestyle after Bariatric Surgery

Your Onederland | The Bariatric Surgery Squad

Acknowledgement

The road to become your best self isn't the easy way out. You made a lifelong commitment when you chose bariatric surgery. And there's no looking back. When you decide it's time for a drastic change, you have to wake up with a sense of purpose - every single day again. And yes, there are going to be times, when you just want to throw in the towel, thinking: *"Is it really all worth it?"*.

But fighting for your health and happiness, is *never* a waste of effort.

The Bariatric Blueprint is dedicated to all bariatric warriors who woke up one day and said: *"enough is enough"*. And there's nobody in the world we want to acknowledge, but you.

Thank you for picking up this book to learn more and to change your life with even more impact than you already have so far. Thank you for being here.

Disclaimer

This book is made for educational, entertaining and inspirational purposes only and is not intended as personal or medical advice. By reading this document, the reader acknowledges that the information provided in this book is not intended as nutritional, clinical, medical, legal or financial advice. Always consult a licensed specialist before attempting any techniques presented in this book. All effort has been made to provide correct, accurate and up to date information. No warranties of any kind are declared or implied. By reading this document, the reader agrees that under no circumstances the author is responsible for any direct or indirect losses, as a result of the use of information of this document, including but not limited to inaccuracies, omissions or errors of any kind.

The Bariatric Blueprint Gifts

Reading a book is one thing. But taking further action is what showing up for yourself after bariatric surgery truly entails. To help you stay focused, we want to give you our free Bariatric Blueprint bundle, including the:

- Non-scale victory celebration checklist
- Hydration tracker
- Daily habits checklist
- Monthly habit tracker

Scan the QR-code to claim your freebies. Or access them through the link below. Enjoy!

https://youronederland.com/freebies-the-bariatric-blueprint/

Introduction

When we first started showing up for the bariatric community, we had one mission in mind. To help make bariatric journeys work with nutrition strategies and mindset tips. And to create a bariatric community to call home *(our bariatric surgery squad!)*.

We're here to show compassion and to remove the stigma that bariatric surgery still holds in this day and age. Luckily things are improving. Education is getting better and as a cherry on top, obesity is officially labeled a chronic disease opening up new doors for both practitioners and patients in the field of bariatric care.

There's no archetype. But there's tons of research to fall back on. Nobody can predict how you feel once you've had your digestive system surgically altered. But knowing what you can expect, can take away some of the guesswork when you're going through the motions of your post-op life.

Here's a question: when you travel towards an unknown destination, would you rather turn on your GPS knowing which way to go – or would you just start driving "hoping" you'll turn up in the right place?

Having bariatric surgery is like unraveling a blueprint, finding new ways to structure your life afterwards. And while you explore, you're bound to run into a bunch of questions that need answers:

Why do I feel hungry one day, and am completely full the next?

Why does my weight stall suddenly and should I do something about it?

What about hair loss, dumping syndrome and "the foamies?".

What are the facts about oral health and tailbone pain?

And, should I really be that afraid of stretching my stomach?

The Bariatric Blueprint gives you a complete framework of how life after bariatric surgery can look like, and what strategies you need to maintain long-term success.

We shed light on the common and less common events after bariatric surgery. Because understanding the science behind *why* certain things happen in your journey, makes it easier to overcome all obstacles.

The chapters of The Bariatric Blueprint are inspired by the Your Onederland Blog *(also known as "The Bariatric Mini-Guides")*. We bundled our best reads, added more insight, and organized them into 5 parts, so that you can easily navigate through the topics.

Stop dreaming of a new you, instead become that person today. Stop thinking of ways to "be better", but take small steps every day. Never stop trying. You got this!

Your Onederland
The "Bariatric Surgery Squad" that will always be on your side

Content

Part 1

Things you wish someone told you before bariatric surgery

Chapter 1

Why "eating less and moving more" didn't work

Even though the first bariatric surgery procedure dates back to the 1950s, the stigma of weight loss surgery still exists to this day. Shockingly, obesity wasn't even labeled an official disease until 2013. That's just a decade ago.

So, it may not come as a total surprise that there's still a stigma surrounding bariatric surgery as a treatment for obesity, considering the 63-year time gap between the first bariatric procedure and the worldwide acknowledgment for obesity being a chronic disease.

"Just eat less and move more"
"Have you tried this diet already?"
"My neighbors' friend had bariatric surgery and gained all of her weight back"

Statements like these, worsen the stigma around bariatric surgery. Making it somewhat feel like you're "failing" if you decide to have your stomach surgically altered instead of "doing it on your own".

But here's the thing.

Obesity is a chronic disease with many underlying factors that go far beyond the sheer act of willpower alone.

There are hormonal, inflammatory, environmental and genetic variables that are part of the chronic illness that obesity truly is. Also, there may be underlying physical and mental health disorders that amplify these factors.

For instance, someone with insulin resistance may crave more simple sugars or more high-caloric foods, because the body reacts differently to the metabolization of glucose. And somebody who is suffering from depression, may crave more sugar to activate the reward system in the brain releasing more dopamine. Obesity causes chronic stress *(physically and mentally)*, chronic inflammation and often a dysregulated gut microbiome, making it harder to lose weight. If you suffer from obesity, you have to work harder to lose weight, but most of all, keep it off long-term compared to someone who doesn't have obesity.

Here's how to break it down a bit further.

It's harder to lose the weight when you're obese, because there's more weight to lose to get to a healthy body weight in the first place. As you can imagine, it's more manageable to lose 10 pounds as it is to lose 100 pounds. On top of that, hunger and satiety cues are often derailed before bariatric surgery. Research shows, that there's a dysregulation of hunger and satiety hormones making the urge to eat greater and the urge to stop eating, much more challenging.

You get the gist.

It's not as simple as "eat less and move more" when we look at a long-term solution for obesity.

Also, if you've been dieting for years, your metabolism takes a major a hit. Your body may have been in a constant "fight-or-flight" state not knowing when it will go in starvation mode again *(the dieting part)* or when the dieting is "over".

Here, we need to make a distinction between *dieting* or *a fad diet* and *your diet* after bariatric surgery. Dieting refers to the "quick-fixes" to lose weight without taking the overall picture, like obesity, stress, habits, other underlying illnesses and lifestyle factors into account. Diets only focus on the outcome by facilitating a calorie deficit which results in weight loss. To worsen the simplicity of a fad diet, they often fail to make a distinction between weight loss *(muscles, water and fat)* or fat loss *(the long-term effective way of losing weight)*. Furthermore, diets have not been designed to be maintained long-term, resulting in weight gain, time and time again.

Your diet after bariatric surgery refers to your eating habits as part of an overall lifestyle change, to keep up with in the long run. The aim now, is a change in lifestyle. Going back to the vicious cycle of dieting, isn't part of the solution after bariatric surgery.

The fact that diets don't work long-term, is backed by research that shows that up to 95% of diets indeed do not result in weight loss maintenance long-term. That's more than 9 out of 10 attempts to lose weight down the drain. That's more than 9 out of 10 people getting their hopes up, just to have them crushed again when the weight trickles back up.

So, it's time to fully acknowledge that a medical treatment is an effective method to treat obesity. And of course, here's where bariatric surgery chimes in.

Chapter takeaways

- Obesity is a complex disease with many underlying factors making it harder to lose weight and maintain weight loss with conservative methods, like dieting and exercise alone.
- Diets don't work long-term. They don't support sustainable weight loss.
- Bariatric surgery is an effective treatment to treat obesity, along with lifestyle interventions and continuous follow-up care.

Chapter 2

3 Myths about bariatric surgery

Now, to fully emerge in the strategies and breakdowns that The Bariatric Blueprint has to offer, let's clear up some myths first. We have to address 3 common myths about bariatric surgery so that you move through the chapters without the judgment that may linger from society, "friends" or even family members who intentionally or unintentionally made you feel like you made the wrong decision to change your life through bariatric surgery.

Because the harsh truth is this: not everyone will be supportive of your decision to go forward with bariatric surgery. And some people may even try to make you feel bad about it. We hope that we can be a beacon of reassurance and a blanket of kindness, making the harsh blows of (unspoken) judgment you have had to endure in the past, a bit softer.

Let's start with the first misconception: *bariatric surgery is dangerous.*

Myth #1 Bariatric surgery is dangerous

It goes without saying that every single surgery has risks. And bariatric surgery is no exception. Examples of complications that can arise after bariatric surgery are leakage, bowel obstruction, gallstones and (hiatal) hernia.

The mortality rate of bariatric surgery is around 0.1% which is considered low-risk. And the likelihood of major complications after bariatric surgery is around 4%.

Although bariatric surgery may not be the right treatment for everyone who is suffering from obesity *(that's because contra indications such as binge eating disorder or sever substance abuse, can interfere with post-op safety and positive outcomes)*, the numbers don't lie.

According to the data gathered by the *American Society for Metabolic and Bariatric Surgery (ASMBS)*, "bariatric surgery leads to 60% of excess weight loss six months after surgery, and 77% of excess weight loss as early as 12 months after surgery. On average, five years after surgery, patients maintain 50% of their excess weight loss".

But bariatric surgery is not about weight loss alone. Treating obesity often goes hand-in-hand with treating its co-morbidities too, like type 2 diabetes, hypertension and cardiovascular disease.

The (temporary) resolution of these so-called co-morbidities is impressive to say the least. We call these the remission rates. Keep in mind that obesity is a chronic disease, which means that it's very much possible that either obesity itself or its co-morbidities can return in time, if the disease of obesity is not controlled any longer *(for example, when helpful lifestyle changes are neglected or post-operative follow up support is lacking)*.

Here are a handful of remission rates that show the effectiveness of bariatric surgery:

Table 1. Remission rates in light of conditions associated with obesity *(ASMBS statistics)*

Condition	Remission Rate
Type 2 Diabetes	92%
Hypertension	75%
Obstructive Sleep Apnea	96%
Dyslipidemia	76%
Cardiovascular Disease	58%

Keep in mind that the risks of not treating obesity often outweigh the risks of bariatric surgery. With that being said, it's of **utmost importance** to commit to:

1. The guidelines from your surgeon's center.
2. Counseling with a therapist for unraveling psychological trauma that have led to a disturbed relationship with food, if applicable.
3. Regular blood work as advised by your surgeon or healthcare provider to detect nutritional

deficiencies in time and making sure your blood work is up to par.

4. Continued follow-up care over the many post-op years that follow.

And this brings us right to the second myth about bariatric surgery.

Myth #2 Bariatric surgery is the easy way out

First, we have to address something. Just because people say or think it's the easy way out, doesn't mean that you owe them an explanation of any kind. But we do need to bring this myth to light, to empower you in your decision for bariatric surgery. So that you know for a fact that you didn't take a "short-cut".

Bariatric surgery comes with a plethora of guidelines. And it starts in the very pre-operative stage, where you first need to get qualified for surgery itself.

During the pre-op stage your calendar may be jam-packed with nutritional appointments, psychology evaluations, sleep study tests, lab-tests *(for example to rule out a Helicobacter Pylori infection)* and of course the kick-off of your liver shrinking diet.

Just the road to surgery alone isn't easy. And the hardest part is yet to come: navigating your post-operative life. Although of course, losing weight often leads to an overall improvement in quality of life. But there are also side-effects, unexplained events and issues that you may experience afterwards. And it's not just the physical effects, like dumping syndrome or constipation, that you may be burdened with. We're talking about the mindset changes too. A new way of eating, eating out in public, how weight loss affects the relationship with others around you, not being able to use food as the same coping mechanism as before surgery and the list goes on.

If anything, bariatric surgery is not the easy way out. Oftentimes, it's the *only* way out. The only way to tackle obesity. And the only way to live life to the fullest, instead of watching it go by from the sidelines.

Myth #3 You have to eat 800-1000 calories for the rest of your life

Bariatric surgery brings you in a calorie deficit as the size of your stomach is reduced. This means your portions decrease too. But you're not meant to eat the smallest amount of food forever. And being in such an extreme calorie deficit, isn't only unsustainable, it can be dangerous too.

Malnourishment is a risk after bariatric surgery due to stomach size reduction and malabsorption in mixed procedures like the gastric bypass.

It's not the goal to eat as less as you can. The goal is to create a healthy relationship with food, while focusing on staying well-nourished in combination with a life-long vitamin regime.

Bariatric surgery isn't about losing weight fast. It's about creating habits that last. Don't be surprised when you're able to eat more as time passes. We'll go into further detail of fluctuating appetite in Chapter 9.

But how many calories should you eat then?

The answer is: it depends.

It depends on how much energy you personally need. And the amount of energy you need is dependent on different variables, such as your basal metabolic rate (BMR), your muscle mass and how much energy you use in the form of physical activity. For example, the more muscle mass you have, the higher your BMR and the more calories you may need. Also, if you have an active lifestyle, you'll need more energy as opposed to having a sedentary lifestyle.

Chapter takeaways

- The myths about bariatric surgery reinforce the stigma surrounding obesity and surgical options to treat it.
- Debunking myths is a necessary step to tackle misinformation and to spread proper education to remove judgment in today's society when it comes down to obesity and bariatric surgery.
- Common myths are: bariatric surgery is dangerous, it's the easy way out and you can only eat a small number of calories for the rest of your life.

Chapter 3

How to prepare for bariatric surgery

Although nobody can really prepare you for the roller coaster ride after bariatric, there are a few things you can do, to give yourself a head start in your journey.

Besides checking off your mandatory pre-op appointments, you can also actively start preparing for your "big day" at home. Already had bariatric surgery? Don't skip this chapter!

Instead, read the tips and check-in with yourself: How did my journey change? Am I still focused on the basic principles that help me move forward?

Focus on high-protein meals

Protein is the key macronutrient after bariatric surgery.

Learning which food sources are high in protein and which ones aren't, gives more clarity to plan and prep your meals. One thing to keep in mind here, is that your taste buds may change once you had bariatric surgery. Not all foods that you enjoy now, will give you the same satisfaction after bariatric surgery.

But how do you get that protein-oriented mindset before surgery? Where to begin? Let's show you how.

3 Tips to create more focus around protein

1. Make food lists with your favorite high-protein food sources *(use the list in Chapter 6 for more inspiration)*.
2. Find new recipes using your food list from the previous tip.
3. Make a meal plan for the day so that you can meet your protein goals better. Talk to your dietitian or surgeon to find out which protein recommendations are right for you. General guidelines state that bariatric patients should consume at least 60-80 grams protein daily. Individual needs may differ.

Focus on staying hydrated

Staying hydrated after bariatric surgery can be a strenuous task. And here's why:

- High restriction means limited intake of food. This also makes it harder to drink liquids.
- You're not able to drink together with your meals.
- The taste of plain water may make you nauseous after bariatric surgery.
- Bariatric surgery requires a limitation in high-sugar beverages leaving out options such as concentrated fruit juice or high-sugar sodas. In other words, you have to get creative with adding more flavor to your water.

Working on your hydration goals *before* you have surgery, will make it more manageable to keep up with hydration afterwards. If you get into a hydration-routine now, you reap the benefits later.

The secret of nourishment: small frequent meals

When you're left with about 20% of your stomach, it's going to be so much more challenging to get all your nutrients in. So, what strategy do you need to make sure you're nourished?

The answer is having small nutrient-dense meals, multiple times a day.

The rule of thumb is usually to have 5-8 small meals daily. But these recommendations can differ from person to person. You may be fulfilled with 5 meals daily. Perhaps you can't eat more often than 3 times a day. Or maybe you need a couple of more "eating moments" to feel satisfied, while also hitting your nutrition goals. Working 1:1 with a dietitian in the pre-op stage, luckily, is often mandatory so that you can figure out what works best for you.

Be aware of the comparison trap

The bariatric community is grand, diverse and unique. Just like any other community there's the good, the bad and the ugly. You can find tons of support and wonderful resources. There are many people who share their process and progress online and you may feel inspired watching their journeys unfold. But there's one thing that can wreak havoc on your peace of mind.

And that is *the comparison trap.*

When you fall for the comparison trap it takes away from you own focus. In Chapter 15 we give you the details on how to break the comparison trap after bariatric surgery.

Find your people, both professionally and personally

This may seem obvious, but don't be mistaken. Not everybody gets the support they deserve on a silver platter. You may have to actively look for a supportive community in order to feel secure and connected to others who understand you. And to those who can help you professionally too.

When your whole life is about to change, it's necessary to have the right people in your corner. People that support you. People that give you solid advice. Friends and family who are there for you, no matter what. A bariatric community that will never let you down *(find free bariatric support groups on www.community.youronederland.com)*.

Take a close look at your bariatric team and check to see if you need more help. Could you benefit from a therapist? Would it be helpful to hire a personal trainer? Are you looking for someone to guide you spiritually? You're the one who knows best what's right for you.

And never forget that investing in your own health, is never a waste of time.

Identify non-hunger cues

Now is the time to start working on your relationship with food if you haven't done so already. Eating is so much more than grabbing a plate, stick the food on a fork and eat it.

Eating is emotional too. All eating-triggers that aren't related to physical hunger are called "non-hunger cues". They can be activated by a specific environment *(for example, a party with lots of food displayed)* or by people *(for example, your "food buddies")*.

Here are 3 examples of non-hunger cues:

- Certain emotions can trigger (over)eating, such as sadness
- Stress can easily lead to poor food choices and/or (over)eating
- Specific environments may trigger (over)eating behavior

Also, it can be challenging to be fully aware of the difference between *mind hunger* or *physical hunger*. Especially if you've been on the "dieting bandwagon" for ages and you're struggling with disrupted eating behaviors such as emotional eating or food addiction.

On top of that, research shows that bariatric patients have a hard time reading their hunger and fullness cues, even *before* bariatric surgery.

Our best tips? Make a list of the reasons why you (over)eat. And ask for psychological guidance if you need to. Bariatric resizes your stomach and changes your hunger hormones. But it doesn't fix any root causes of emotional eating, self-sabotaging behaviors or other disrupted eating patterns. And this is the hard part. This is the part that is often overlooked: the mindset work that is required to start, and most of all, maintain your habits for life *(we'll get into the depth of creating new habits in Chapter 17).*

Ditch the 'all-or-nothing' mindset

All-or-nothing thinking is also referred to as black and white thinking. This distorted way of perceiving reality, supports the false belief that there are only two outcomes: success or failure. There's no room for a gray area with all-or-nothing thinking: it's a fixed mindset.

An all-or-nothing mindset is an unhelpful coping mechanism in the light of sustaining new habits. It doesn't allow any nuances and thus, severely restricts your ability to move forward after bariatric surgery.

To give you an idea, here are a handful of examples you may recognize yourself:

"There are only good and bad foods"
"If I don't lose 2 pounds by the end of the week, I'm not successful"

"My weight is stalling; I must be doing something wrong"
"I gained 3 pounds; I messed it up"
"I will never succeed"
"If I don't follow my plan today, I'm a bad bariatric patient"
"If I don't prep my meals today, I won't succeed"

The all-or-nothing mindset is part of a fixed mindset, making it harder to grow. Being aware of these thought processes is the first step to changing them.

In Chapter 16 we give you a more in-depth strategy to get rid of the all-or-nothing mentality after bariatric surgery.

Chapter takeaways

- Nobody can truly prepare you for everything that's bound to happen in your bariatric journey.
- Preparing within the realms of reality, is necessary to get used to new habits.
- Strategies to prepare for bariatric surgery are: focusing on protein and hydration, having small frequent meals, finding support for the long run and bringing mindset challenges – like the all-or-nothing mindset – to light.

Chapter 4

9 Things nobody talks about before bariatric surgery

In this Chapter, we want to create awareness about 9 events that you may not have heard (enough) about before you started your journey. Maybe you're experiencing some of these lesser-known side-effects right now. Keep in mind, that not everybody has the same physical response to bariatric surgery. But being aware of what potentially could happen, can give more reassurance when it does.

#1 Regurgitation of food: The foamies

The foamies is referred to as the regurgitation of mucus and undigested small food particles that move back up from your stomach, into your mouth. The foamies is also known as *"foamy mouth"*.

The foamies can happen when:

- you eat too fast
- you don't chew thoroughly
- food doesn't sit well in your stomach

And what anatomically happens is this:

The opening between your stomach and your small intestine *(called the stoma in mixed procedures)* is blocked by the food that's inside your stomach, which makes it nearly impossible for your food to pass through during this moment. Your stomach produces more mucus in order for the food to pass, but the exact opposite may happen: the food and mucus regurgitates.

The best way to prevent the foamies, is to eat slow and chew well. But even if you're eating mindful, you may still be caught by surprise by the nauseating slime in the back of your throat.

#2 Struggling with bowel movements: Constipation

The first few days after bariatric surgery can be pretty rough. You're still trying to figure out how to eat, drink and not to mention – to get rid of the gas pain.

Constipation may be at its peak in the first weeks after bariatric surgery. The good news is, that bowel movements should slowly improve over the following 6 months post-op. However, medication, diet and physical activity can impact your bowel health differently.

So, why is constipation more common after bariatric surgery?

Main reasons for post-op constipation may be:

- lack of fiber

- lack of hydration
- lack of exercise
- medication
- supplements such as iron or calcium

As your food intake and food tolerance increases, and you're able to get more fiber and water in, your bowel movements usually improve on its own. Always consult your doctor if you continue to struggle with constipation *(or any other bowel issues for that matter)*.

#3 When you can't unsee the "old you": Body distortion

Bariatric surgery can cause (symptoms) of body dysmorphia, because your brain doesn't seem to be catching up with the rapid weight loss transformation that follows. And this creates a 'mismatch' in how you perceive yourself versus the actual reality.

Symptoms of body dysmorphia are:

- Constantly comparing yourself to others
- Avoiding mirrors – or being overly obsessed with looking in the mirror
- Always asking others for validation about your appearance
- Not being able to accept compliments about your appearance from others
- Hiding (parts of) your body constantly

Keep in mind that *body dysmorphia* is an official DSM-5 disorder that can only be diagnosed by a licensed specialist. Showing signs of body dysmorphia doesn't automatically indicate that you *have* body dysmorphia.

Nevertheless, these feelings shouldn't be underestimated. Because the physical transformation that can happen rapidly after weight loss surgery, has a major impact on how you perceive yourself.

When you don't recognize yourself in the mirror: Body distortion

Body distortion is not uncommon after bariatric surgery and can have serious implications for your mental health. Your body changes rapidly in a short period of time and you may be dealing with excess skin.

Here are 2 tips to help you work through body distortion:

1. Take many before pictures to have a clear visual of the actual difference between "then" and "now". Visuals can minimize the mismatch occurring in your perception.
2. Confide in a therapist to get 1:1 guidance, personalized to your own needs.

Body distortion may present itself throughout different stages after bariatric surgery, as this is different from situation to situation. Don't hesitate to reach out for guidance, if you continue to struggle mentally with how you feel in a "new" body.

#4 Sensitization of the *vagus nerve*: Fullness cues

There are 12 cranial nerves in your nervous system that are involved in sending feedback to your brain from other parts of the body. The *vagus nerve* is the 10th nerve and is the longest one of them all.

Bariatric surgery increases the sensitivity of your vagus nerve. And this could result in new fullness cues, you never experienced before bariatric surgery. Fullness cues are signals to let you know that you're approaching satiety.

These so-called fullness cues can look like this:

- Coughing
- Sighing
- Burping
- Yawning
- Sneezing
- Runny nose

Paying attention to these cues can help you stop eating in time, to keep overeating and digestive issues at bay.

#5 When you regret having bariatric Surgery: "Buyer's remorse"

When you're in agony because of excruciating gas pain while tackling mind hunger and also struggle to get your protein and liquids in – it's not uncommon to experience *buyer's remorse* shortly after bariatric surgery.

Buyer's remorse is referred to as feeling regretful of having bariatric surgery, experienced in the first weeks after your procedure. For most, these feelings pass as you start to heal and you get used to your new normal. If you continue to feel bad about your decision, there are a few things you can do.

First, talking to others who've gone through a similar experience, can be reassuring. Second, don't hesitate to reach out to your bariatric team if you continue to struggle. They're there to provide you with professional guidance. Last, remember that these feelings are likely to pass. Buyer's remorse is often short lived and fades as you start to feel better.

#6 Tailbone pain after bariatric surgery

A lesser-known side-effect of bariatric surgery *(or actually, as a result of losing a significant amount of weight in general)*, is tailbone pain.

The medical name for tailbone pain is *coccydynia*.

When you lose weight after bariatric surgery, you lose fat too. As a result, the padding surrounding your tailbone also decreases. The rubbing of your tailbone against nearby tissue can cause (severe) pain.

Some bariatric patients may find relief by using a special cushion or changing positions often when sitting behind a desk. Always talk to your doctor for personal guidance.

#7 Oral health and the impact of bariatric surgery

There are two reasons why bariatric surgery *(and the eating habits that follow)* can negatively affect your oral health.

First, eating and drinking more frequently, can wreak havoc on your enamel. But the second cause, has a more dramatic impact: tooth decay and tooth loss due to calcium resorption.

You see, when your calcium levels are low *(which can easily happen if you're not consistently taking your calcium supplements and it's challenging to stay nourished)*, your body automatically tries to "find" calcium sources other than the foods you consume.

Your bones and teeth both contain calcium bonds. So, whenever you're experiencing a shortage in calcium, your body has clever ways to restore its balance by snatching away calcium from your bones and teeth. This, in turn, can lead to mineral loss from your teeth and a higher risk of tooth decay and tooth loss.

Talk to your dentist if you had bariatric surgery or preparing for surgery to find a long-term solution.

#8 Loud gurgling sounds from your stomach

Don't be surprised when your stomach suddenly makes the loudest of noises after bariatric surgery. The way that air is being pushed through your stomach is different now, which can cause an orchestra of gurgling sounds.

And there's nothing to completely prevent this, other than making sure that you're not ingesting too much air when you're chewing your food.

#9 The risk of gallstones

Gallstones are hardened parts of bile that are formed in the gallbladder. Bile is a digestive fluid produced by the liver and stored in the gallbladder. Bile helps to digest fats into fatty acids. Bariatric surgery increases the risk of developing gallstones by 10-38%. And the trigger is extremely rapid weight loss or an excessive reduction in weight. It's important to note that obesity already increased the risk of gallstones before bariatric surgery.

Studies also show that women may be at greater risk of developing gallstones than men. Additionally, type of surgery may play a role in the chances of developing gallstones where the gastric bypass seems to lead to a greater risk of gallstones than the gastric sleeve for example *(this doesn't mean that you will develop gallstones if you have the gastric bypass or that you won't develop gallstones if you have the gastric sleeve)*.

Some surgeons will propose preventive strategies, like gallbladder removal or medication, like *ursodeoxycholic acid.*

Gallstones are usually treated by removing the gallbladder altogether.

Chapter takeaways

- Being aware of the lesser-known side-effects of bariatric surgery can help to minimize the surprise for when it happens.
- Some of these side-effects include, but are not exhaustive to, the foamies, gallstones, tailbone pain and a decline in oral health.
- Medical conditions should always be discussed with a healthcare provider.

Chapter 5

What you should know about hair loss

When Delilah was involved in setting up a trap to cut off Samson's hair, something tragic happened. He lost all of his strength and his life turned into misery.

Hair loss after bariatric surgery may not lead to such a biblical tragedy. However, it can have a pretty negative impact on your mental well-being.

Research shows that up to 57% of bariatric patients may experience hair loss within the first year after bariatric surgery.

And in this chapter, we explain what the underlying causes may be. But first, let's start with the essence of it all: what does the hair growth process look like?

First things first: The process of hair growth explained

Hair grows in four different stages, which are called the *anagen stage*, the *catagen stage*, the *telogen stage* and the *exogen stage*. The anagen stage is referred to as the cycle in which your hair is actually growing.

On average, about 90% of your hair follicles reside in the anagen stage in any given time and this may last up to 3-5 years.

The catagen stage is a transitional stage between the anagen stage and the telogen stage. In the catagen stage, your body receives the signal that the end of the growth-phase approaches. The catagen stage lasts around 10 days and about 2-3% of your hair resides in that stage at any given time.

Moving on, we're approaching the telogen stage where your hair isn't actively growing, but remains attached to its follicles. You have entered the resting stage of hair growth. And about 10-15% of your hair resides in this stage at any given time.

The last stage of your hair growth cycle is called the exogen stage. And as the name already implies, refers to your hair falling out so that the process can start from scratch. Now, you may be tempted to believe that hair loss after bariatric surgery occurs in the exogen stage of the hair growth cycle. But this isn't the case.

You see, when you shed hair naturally the exogen phase is where we stand. But if we look at hair loss after bariatric surgery, the event takes place in an earlier stage of the hair growth cycle. That's why holding the clumps of hair after taking a shower, comes as an unpleasant surprise. Telogen effluvium refers to losing hair during the telogen stage of the hair growth cycle *(the phase where your hair is 'resting' from growth).*

The big question remains yet to be answered:

"Is it possible to prevent hair loss after bariatric surgery? And if so, what can you do about it?"

Before we dive into that question, let's explain some of the main (hypothesized) causes for hair loss after bariatric surgery.

Reasons for hair loss after bariatric surgery unraveled: Nutritional and non-nutritional

Not all causes of hair loss are completely explained in relation to your diet. There are a few hypothesis in clinical research that explain some of the reasons for post-operative hair loss beyond the scope of what's on your plate.

Like mentioned before, up to 57% of bariatric patients experience hair loss within the first year after bariatric surgery. Most hair loss occurs around the 3-4 month post-op mark and may last around 6 months before it starts growing back. Keep in mind that these outcomes are different for each and every individual or situation! Nobody can truly predict what will happen to you personally.

Here are 3 things to keep in mind when looking at non-nutritional causes for hair loss:

- Bariatric surgery in itself is a stressful event for your body. The stress that's triggered may cause hair to fall out.
- Bariatric surgery brings you in a so-called *catabolic state*. This means that your body is in full force "breakdown-mode". This catabolic state can cause hair to fall out too.
- Bariatric surgery may inflict stress mentally. Keeping up with the guidelines and pivoting around a whole new way of eating, is stressful to say the least. This type of stress is assumed to be related to early onset hair loss as well.

What stands out if you look at the 3 reasons above? That's right. They're beyond your control. You can't control the physical stress that bariatric surgery brings. And you can't control the catabolic state of your body neither. This is why it's important to emphasize that hair loss isn't entirely preventable.

You can't blame yourself for post-op hair loss, but it is important to *be aware* of what role nutrition plays in keeping your hair as healthy as possible. To do that, we have to take a closer look at four nutrients that are related to hair loss after bariatric surgery.

The quality of your food matters: protein, zinc, ferritin and folic acid

There's a broad spectrum of research that looks into nutritional hair loss after bariatric surgery. Simply put:

studies are trying to answer the question which nutrients are related to hair loss after bariatric surgery. And here are some interesting findings that are directly related to the foods you eat, the vitamins you take and of course in mixed procedures – the degree of malabsorption. Keep in mind that individual needs differ, and ones personal guidelines should always be discussed with a (para)medical health care professional like a surgeon or a dietitian.

Protein and nutritional hair loss

One of the symptoms of a protein deficiency is hair loss. The majority of bariatric patients does not meet their protein goals, even in the long-term when restriction decreases. Here's a quick glance of high protein food sources:

- Meat, poultry, fish and other seafood
- Eggs
- Yogurt, (butter)milk and quark
- (Cottage) cheese
- Legumes and pulses
- Nuts, nut butters and seeds
- Protein supplements like protein powders, protein shakes and protein bars

General guidelines state that 60-80 grams of protein daily is the minimum requirement after bariatric surgery. Spreading your meals evenly throughout the day and making sure you eat your protein first, increases the chance that you'll hit your protein goals.

The role of zinc in nutritional hair loss after bariatric surgery

Zinc is a mineral that has different meaningful functions in your body like:

- Supporting the immune system
- Cell growth and cell division
- The synthesis of DNA
- Supporting different enzyme functions

According to the general guidelines, zinc requirements differ based on type of bariatric procedure and may vary between 8-22 milligrams daily. A zinc deficiency is directly related to hair loss after bariatric surgery. So here's two things you can be mindful of:

1. Take your vitamins as prescribed to you
2. Include foods that are naturally high in zinc

Foods that are high in zinc:

- Oysters
- Other seafood
- Red meat
- Poultry
- Legumes
- Nuts & seeds

Folic acid and hair loss after bariatric surgery

Not only do pregnant women benefit from folic acid during their first trimester especially, bariatric patients do too. You see, a folic acid deficiency increases the likelihood of hair loss. The general requirements for folic acid are 400-800 micrograms from a daily vitamin and 800-1000 micrograms from a daily vitamin for women of childbearing age. Again, personal recommendations may differ.

And if you're wondering whether you're eating the right foods that contain folic acid, here's list of high folic acid foods to remember:

- Asparagus
- Eggs
- Dark leafy vegetables
- Brussel sprouts
- Broccoli
- Beans
- Beets
- Citrus fruits

Ferritin and hair loss after bariatric surgery

Now we hear you thinking, what's the difference between iron and ferritin?

Let's explain.

Ferritin is a protein that resides in your blood and stores iron. Perhaps you're familiar with a ferritin test to detect an iron deficiency. When your ferritin levels are low, you don't have enough iron stored in your body. Hence, your iron levels are low too.

An iron deficiency can occur after bariatric surgery due to malabsorption and food intolerances towards high-iron food sources.

Foods that are high in iron, are often foods that aren't tolerated well any longer. Take red meat for example. Red meat is high in iron, but often much more difficult to digest once you had bariatric surgery.

On top of that, we also have to make a distinction between heme iron *(found in animal-based products, heme iron is easier absorbed)* and non-heme iron *(found in plant-based products, non-heme iron is more difficult to absorb)*. This shows that it's not always as easy to "stay nourished" after bariatric surgery.

One nutritional "hack" to make sure you're absorbing your iron to the maximum, is to combine iron-rich foods and foods that are high in vitamin C together. For example, when you eat ground beef *(high in iron)*, combine this with broccoli *(high in vitamin C)*. What you want to avoid as much as possible is taking high-calcium foods in combination with high-iron foods. Also, food that contains *tannins*, like tea, can hinder iron absorption.

Chapter takeaways

- Hair loss after bariatric surgery is often temporary.
- Hair loss can be the cause of non-nutritional factors, such as stress and the body's catabolic state after bariatric surgery.
- Hair loss can have nutritional causes, of which protein, zinc, folic acid and ferritin are a handful of nutrients to pay close attention to.

Part 2

How to nail the bariatric guidelines

Chapter 6

Understanding nutrition and maximizing your protein intake

Bariatric surgery challenges you in many ways. You have to take on a whole new way of eating, starting as early as the pre-operative liquid diet to shrink the size of your liver. But it doesn't stop there.

After surgery, you have to follow the postoperative-diet in which you slowly, and in consultation with your bariatric care team, introduce new foods and textures back to your diet.

Once you can tolerate most, if not all, foods, you may find out that you're able to eat more than you used to. A normal part of eating after bariatric surgery. Let's call this: *portion progression.*

While protein is the first macronutrient to focus on after bariatric surgery, ultimately, it's the goal to include a wide variety of nutrients in due time. Let's call this: *nutrient progression.*

Keep in mind that eating after bariatric surgery isn't tied to one specific strategy only. Your appetite, restriction and therefore your portions fluctuate throughout your journey. This may even be the case many years later.

The pre-operative diet

The diet prior to your surgery date is also known as the liver shrinking diet or the liver reduction diet. This diet is meant to reduce the size of your liver before surgery. Reducing liver size lowers the risk of bleeding during the surgery procedure. Having a smaller liver increases the likelihood of your surgery being more successful *(less complications, clears operation site)*.

Guidelines regarding the pre-operative diet differ from surgeon to surgeon, but they all have one thing in common: low-calorie, low-fat and high-protein. Some patients start the pre-operative diet 2 weeks before surgery, while others just 2 days before their surgery.

The post-operative diet

Right after surgery, you need time to recover. Your new stomach is still swollen and there's barely space. Together with your surgeon or dietitian you discuss a post-operative diet plan to slowly progress from liquids to solid foods in the upcoming weeks after your surgery.

The guidelines regarding the post-operative diet, just like the pre-operative diet, vary from surgeon to surgeon. But they typically have 5 different phases, of which the daily recommended intake of protein is 60-80 grams and liquids 64 ounces. Keep in mind that you may not hit those targets right after bariatric surgery, but the goal is to stay hydrated and focus on your protein, so that your recovery progress goes as smooth as possible. Here are the 5 different phases of the post-operative diet:

Stage 1 Clear Liquids
The main purpose of the first stage is to keep you well hydrated right after surgery. You'll have to take small sips throughout the day. Examples of clear liquids are: water and clear broth.

Stage 2 Full Liquids
Some surgeons will skip the full liquid stage and move straight to the puréed stage. Examples of high-protein full liquids are: skim milk, strained cream soups and protein shakes.

Stage 3 Puréed Foods
For many, moving forward to the puréed stage is exciting to say the least. You've missed the taste of 'real food' and you're looking forward to have more variety. Foods eaten in the puréed stage should all be blended until smooth.

Stage 4 Soft Foods
You're gradually moving on to more solid foods and the stabilization diet. Sometimes you have to move back to a previous stage if any complications occur. Examples of high-protein soft foods are: white fish, low-fat yogurt, eggs and cottage cheese.

Stage 5 Solid Foods
As you enter the final stage of the post-op diet, you're slowly introducing a wider variety of foods. Maybe you're

intolerant to certain foods. Important habits to remember are: keeping solids from liquids, chewing your food thoroughly and eating your protein first.

The main focus right after surgery are protein and hydration. Dehydration is one of the main reasons for re-admittance after bariatric surgery, and is not to be underestimated. More strategies on how to stay hydrated are listed in Chapter 7.

Protein after bariatric surgery

Protein is one of the macronutrients along with carbohydrates and fat. Protein consists of building blocks, called the amino acids. In total, there are 20 amino acids of which 9 of those your body isn't able to make on its own. These are called the essential amino acids and need to be derived from your diet. The other 11 amino acids can be produced by your body. And these are called, not surprisingly, the non-essential amino acids.

Now, let's explain why protein is such an important nutrient after bariatric surgery.

1. You need protein to preserve your muscle mass

Protein is what your muscles are made of. Without protein, you're not only skimping on building muscles, but you're at a much higher risk of actually losing muscle mass too.

We hear you thinking: *"But I really don't want to build any muscles, do I still need protein?"*

The answer to that question is a firm yes!

And by sufficient protein intake through your diet and incorporating (light) resistance training, you can minimize muscle loss.

2. Protein promotes physical recovery

A high-protein diet speeds up the physical recovery process after any surgery. And bariatric surgery isn't an exception. The hurdle is that with a smaller stomach and immediate digestive issues like nausea, it's more challenging to keep up with the daily protein recommendations right off the bat.

It's common sense to rely on protein shakes in the early stages to meet your protein targets. Over time, solid foods will replace most protein shakes *(but, it's also quite common to still need protein shakes every now and then, whenever your restriction is too high to consume dense protein food sources or you're suffering from digestive issues).*

3. Protein helps to curb appetite

Protein is dense and helps to stabilize your blood sugar levels too. It takes longer to digest a high-protein meal, than a meal high in refined sugars for example.

This means that protein keeps you full longer. Also, a high-protein diet is associated with a decrease in appetite.

So not only does protein help with muscle mass maintenance and healing, it also helps to keep cravings in check.

The "Protein Catch-22"

If you ever wondered, why it's easier to eat a bowl of chips than to finish 3 pieces of chicken, then let's talk about the *(as we like to call it)* "catch-22" of meeting your protein goals after bariatric surgery.

Let's explain.

Foods that are high in protein, are often more filling too, because protein is dense. On one hand, this works wonders for suppressing certain cravings. Protein helps to curb your appetite this way, remember? But on the other hand, it can also be a pitfall when your restriction is already high.

In other words: if you're already struggling to eat a proper meal without feeling full after just one bite, it's going to be so much more challenging to meet your protein requirements every day.

If you're feeling overwhelmed right now with the task to eat your protein without feeling sick to your stomach, then let's quickly move on to 5 ways to meet your protein goals better.

Protein Strategy #1 – Know your high-protein food sources

Eating enough protein, all starts with being aware of which foods are high in protein and which ones aren't.

So, here's a quick protein list to help you decide which foods you want to add to your diet. Use this as inspiration for your own meals and snacks. A quick hack to remember is this: every 1 ounce (28 grams) of a lean protein food source, has about 7 grams of protein. So, if you have 3 ounces of chicken breast, this would add up to about 21 grams of protein in total.

High-Protein Food Sources:

1. Lean meats and poultry
- Chicken
- Turkey
- Lean (ground) beef
- Lean cuts of pork

2. Fish and seafood
- Cod
- Trout
- Halibut
- Shrimp
- Scallop
- Salmon
- Mackerel
- Herring

3. Dairy and eggs
- Cottage cheese
- (Greek) yogurt
- Quark
- Milk
- Buttermilk
- Other cheese

4. Legumes and pulses
- All beans
- Lentils
- Chickpeas
- Black eyed peas

5. Nuts and seeds
- Almonds
- Walnuts
- Cashews
- Peanuts
- Pistachios
- Hemp seed
- Chia seed

6. Soy products
- Edamame beans
- Soy beans
- Tofu
- Tempeh

Dairy contains protein. But there's a caveat when it comes down to dairy after bariatric surgery. You see, bariatric surgery increases the likelihood of lactose intolerance. Especially after mixed procedures like the gastric bypass, where absorption in the small intestine is compromised.

Here's how this works.

The enzyme responsible for the breakdown of lactose is called *lactase*. After bariatric surgery, lactase may become less available to help you digest high-lactose foods, such as milk and cream.

If you become lactose-intolerant, you may not be able to tolerate dairy any longer. And you guessed it, you'll have to focus more on lactose-free food sources to meet your protein goals.

Protein Strategy #2 – Make protein your priority

To make sure that protein is your priority, you have to build your meals around protein.

So instead of having spaghetti with meatballs, think of your meal as "meatballs with spaghetti". That way, you shift the focus on protein being the star player of your dish.

Pick one or maybe even two high-protein food sources, and build your meal from there. A simple method to help you with building your post-op meals, once you're able to add more foods back to your diet, is called "The Bariatric Plate Method". In this method your plate consists of 50%

protein, 30% fruit or non-starchy vegetables and 20% complex carbs. That is, when you're able to tolerate most foods of course.

Protein Strategy #3 – Add protein to your beverage choices

The aim after bariatric surgery is to ultimately eat as "normal" as possible without having to rely on protein shakes to meet your protein goals. But the reality is this: on some days, your restriction may be too high to eat a full plate of solids. Your appetite may fluctuate, even years later, making it challenging sometimes to eat a meal with dense solid protein sources like beef or chicken.

On those days, it can be helpful to get your protein from the "easier" (less solid) protein food sources like:

- Protein shakes
- Greek yogurt
- Quark
- Skim milk
- Cottage cheese (blended)
- Protein water
- Soy milk
- Soy yogurt
- High-protein milk products

The denser protein food sources will help you feel full for longer and include the following:

- Meat, poultry, fish and seafood

- Tofu and tempeh
- Eggs

Choose your protein sources, depending on what you're able to tolerate.

Protein Strategy #4 – Eat your protein *before* you get too full

A fourth strategy to prioritize your protein is to *eat your protein first*. Your restriction *(how much food you're able to consume in one sitting)* can be high after bariatric surgery because of the following reasons:

- Your surgery wasn't too long ago *(the further you're out, usually, the less restricted you feel)*
- You feel stressed
- You're not feeling well overall
- It's just the way your restriction is *(it's personal to your situation)*

Restriction feels different for everyone. There's no right or wrong restriction, there's just *your stomach* and *your restriction*. And how much food you're able to tolerate varies greatly between days, and sometimes between meals even.

By eating your protein first, you make sure that you're not too full.

Protein Strategy #5 – Break down your protein goal into small steps

Let's say that your daily protein goal is 80 grams.

Breaking your daily protein goal into smaller steps can be helpful to lessen the overwhelm.

If you intend on having 3 main meals (breakfast, lunch and dinner) and 3 snacks (morning, afternoon and evening snack) today, this sums up to 6 "eating moments". When we divide those 80 grams of protein in between those 6 meals, making sure the main meals include more protein than your snacks, we can make a schedule like this:

Table 2. Example of protein breakdown with 80 grams of protein in a day

"Eating Moment"	Amount of protein
Breakfast	15 grams
Morning snack	10 grams
Lunch	15 grams
Afternoon snack	10 grams
Dinner	20 grams
Evening snack	10 grams
Total amount of daily protein	**80 grams**

You can tweak this schedule according to your own protein recommendations and the times that you eat normally. Not everyone has the same schedule as this may be affected by your job, your restriction and what you're able to manage in a day.

The key takeaway is to break down your overall goal into small steps. That way, you can simply focus what's in front of you instead of getting lost in the general guidelines.

Carbohydrates after bariatric surgery

Carbohydrates have been presented in a bad light, if we look at *diet culture,* where you may have heard statements like "fruit is bad for you because it has too much sugar" or that you have to "cut out all carbs" to lose weight.

Nutrition after bariatric surgery should <u>not</u> be about going back to restrictive diets that lean into an all-or-nothing way of thinking. Not only are the statements above about carbohydrates false, they often hinder you from rebuilding a healthy relationship with food.

There are two types of carbohydrates *(let's call them carbs from now on).* There are simple carbs, like the ones found in fruit, table sugar and honey. And there are complex carbs, like the ones found in whole grains, legumes and bread. Both simple and complex carbs are broken down by your digestive system *(with the help of an enzyme called amylase)*, into glucose.

Glucose is stored in your body as glycogen, in your muscles and liver. Insulin is the hormone responsible for the transportation of glucose to your cells. Glucagon, also a hormone, helps to release glucose from your cells, to use for energy.

So, it doesn't come as a surprise that your body's main energy source is glucose, derived from the carbs in your diet.

Complex carbs and a handful of simple-carb containing foods such as fruit and some vegetables, are the carbs that are going to be most helpful in your diet after bariatric surgery.

Complex carbs are also the carbs that offer a wider array of nutrients as opposed to the foods that mostly contain refined sugars *(which are simple carbs)*.

As you can see, not all carbs are created equal.

The nutrient diversity in high-carb foods, can vary from a low to a high-range of nutrient diversity.

For example, chocolate chip cookies contain mostly simple carbs in the form of sugar or a sugar derivative. Chocolate chip cookies are also considered a slider food and won't keep you full for long *(more about slider foods in Chapter 12)*. They often lack vitamins and minerals and they're low in fiber too. Not to mention that added sugars, can also increase the risk of dumping syndrome *(more about this side-effect in Chapter 11)*.

In contrast, sweet potatoes *(also a high-carb food source)* offer a range of other helpful nutrients besides the complex carbs in the form of fiber and starch. They're also high in potassium and vitamin C.

These two examples show, that not all carbs are the same. And even within the range of simple and complex carbs, there are differences too – depending on the nutritional value per food source. Also, one is not better than the other. Sometimes, you need simple carbs for a quick boost of energy. But if you're looking for a meal to keep you nourished and full longer, you're better off adding complex carbs to your plate.

To give you a better idea, here are a few examples of foods that are either high in simple or complex carbs.

Table 3. Examples of simple carbohydrates vs complex carbohydrates

Simple Carbohydrates	Complex Carbohydrates
Fruit juice with added sugars	Oatmeal
Soda	Potatoes
Processed foods, like chips and cookies	Whole grain bread
Candy	Brown rice
Ice cream	Legumes like lentils and kidney beans
White bread and pasta	Quinoa

*Fruit and carb-containing vegetables like carrots or sweet peas are an exception to the "simple carb category". These foods contain simple carbs. Yet, they offer a wide array of other helpful nutrients such as fiber, vitamins and minerals. They don't resemble other simple-carb foods such as cookies or chocolate in that sense.

Simple carbs often have a higher glycemic index than complex carbs. Meaning that they raise your blood sugar levels quicker as opposed to the complex carbs as the breakdown into glucose takes more time in complex carbs.

When to add carbs back into your post-op diet

When you just had bariatric surgery and you're still following the post-op diet, you notice that you barely have room to eat your protein, let alone other nutrients like carbs and fat. But the thing is, food is versatile.

For example, split peas are high in protein *and* high in complex carbs. And avocados are high in unsaturated fats *and* in fiber.

Right after surgery, the main focus is protein and hydration, but that doesn't mean that your post-op diet has zero carbs altogether. Working with a dietitian is extremely helpful to make sure that your needs are met.

Foods such as bread, rice or pasta often don't sit well in the new bariatric tummy as they tend to become sticky quickly. Also, they may feel very "heavy" when digested. When to add those type of foods back into your diet depends on your surgeon's advice and what you're able to tolerate. Some people may never get used to eating bread again, while others don't have any issues with bread at all. And the same goes for other high-carb foods such as pasta and rice.

Fats after bariatric surgery

Besides protein and carbs, unsaturated fat plays an important role in your diet as well. Unsaturated fats, such as found in avocados and olive oil may not be suitable right away. Fat can 'sit' more heavily in the post-operative bariatric stomach and cause digestive issues.

However, unsaturated fats are just as much needed after bariatric surgery as they did when you were still pre-op. Foods high in unsaturated fats also contain one or more of the fat-soluble vitamins: A, D, E and K. Besides their high nutritional value, they also help to promote satiety and thus keep you full longer.

In contrast, saturated fats and trans fats are not on the list of "nutrients that your body needs". Does that mean that you have to restrict yourself from certain foods that do contain the unhealthy fats? Not entirely.

You see, bariatric surgery forces you to follow your surgeons' guidelines when you're still healing. But ultimately, bariatric surgery is also about creating a healthy relationship with food. Restricting entire food groups reinforces the all-or-nothing way of thinking and can possibly lead to a more disruptive eating pattern altogether. Of course, the way you choose to handle your relationship with food is entirely up to you. What works for one person, doesn't work for someone else.

Alcohol after bariatric surgery

Does alcohol fit in after bariatric surgery?

It depends.

There are hard guidelines when it comes down to adding alcohol into your diet after bariatric surgery *(common advice is to wait at least 6-12 months after bariatric surgery, but guidelines differ from surgeon to surgeon).* One thing is for certain: alcohol after bariatric surgery goes hand-in-hand with different types of issues.

If we look at (new-onset) alcohol use disorder *(also known as AUD)*, there's conflicting evidence in different studies whether AUD is more common within the bariatric community or not. Some studies suggest that bariatric surgery increases the likelihood of AUD, while other research seems to show no correlation between bariatric surgery and AUD.

Substance use disorders seem to be minimal *(only 1.7%)* when looking at the pre-operative psychological screening data within the bariatric community.

Metabolization of alcohol after bariatric surgery

What we do know is that alcohol is metabolized differently after bariatric surgery, especially after a gastric bypass:

- The absorption of alcohol happens quicker
- There's a higher maximum alcohol concentration
- It takes longer to eliminate alcohol from the body
- There may be an increased risk of AUD *(after a gastric bypass, specifically)*

There's less unanimous data concerning gastric sleeve surgery regarding alcohol absorption. Although, if you are a gastric sleeve patient, you may have experienced first-hand that you:

- Can't tolerate alcohol any longer
- If you do, you feel the "buzz" quicker

Another issue that may arise in the light of alcohol and bariatric surgery, is the increased likelihood of dumping syndrome. Cocktails that are high in sugars, may trigger a dumping episode with ease.

Is alcohol *forbidden* after bariatric surgery? No, it's not. But it's wise to be aware of both physical as well as the emotional consequences of alcohol use after bariatric surgery.

Sadly, transfer addiction is a risk. If food was an addiction before bariatric surgery, or you're having a hard time finding new coping mechanisms besides food after bariatric surgery – it's more likely to experience transfer addiction. A new substance *(in this case it could be alcohol)* is "traded" for the old substance *(food)*.

Micronutrients after bariatric surgery

All vitamins and minerals are considered *micronutrients*. And the numbers don't lie. Micronutrient deficiencies are more common within the bariatric community, starting in the pre-operative stage already. There's evidence that the following nutrients are too low in pre-operative bariatric patients: vitamin D, folic acid, vitamin B1, vitamin B12, vitamin E, zinc, iron and selenium.

Now, bariatric surgery increases the risk of micronutrient deficiencies even more, because of the following reasons:

- Decreased food intake
- Anatomical changes that cause nutrient malabsorption
- Reduction of hydrochloric acid secretion *(stomach acid)* and intrinsic factors *(intrinsic factor is produced in the stomach and necessary to absorb vitamin B12 in the small intestine)*
- Postoperative nausea that results in vomiting *(loss of nutrients)*
- Diarrhea and steatorrhea *(fatty stool, also loss of nutrients)*
- Poor tolerance of specific foods that may provide you with specific nutrients *(for example, if you can't tolerate dairy any longer, it's even more so important to keep a close eye on your calcium intake – as dairy is high in calcium).*

The importance of taking your vitamins every day can't be emphasized enough. But what do the guidelines say? According to the updated guidelines regarding the micronutrients published in 2017 by the ASMBS, these were the recommended nutrient supplementations for post-operative bariatric surgery patients (see table 4 on the next page).

Table 4. Preventive supplements after different bariatric surgery procedures

Nutrients	Gastric Sleeve	Gastric Bypass	Duodenal Switch
Vitamin B1	At least 12 mg/d At risk patients: at least 50-100 mg/d		
Vitamin B12	350–500 ug/d oral, disintegrating tablet, sublingual or liquid – as directed or 1000 mcg/mo intramuscular		
Folate	400-800 mcg oral 800-1000 mcg females childbearing ages		
Calcium	1200-1500 mg/d		1800-2400 mg/d
Vitamin E	15 mg/d		
Vitamin K	90-120 ug/d		300 ug/d
Vitamin D	At least 3000 IU/d to maintain D,25(OH) levels 4 30 ng/mL		
Iron	At least 18 mg/d from multivitamin At least 45–60 mg/d in females with menses and/or patients with history of anemia		
Zinc	8–11 mg/d	8–11 mg/d to 16–22 mg/d	16–22 mg/d

Always discuss your personal micronutrient needs with your healthcare provider.

9 Facts about vitamins to always remember:

1. Calcium citrate is better absorbed than calcium carbonate.

2. Calcium supplements are usually divided into 3 dosages of 500 mg (taken at breakfast, lunch and dinner).
3. Vitamin C can help with iron absorption.
4. Calcium inhibits iron absorption and it's not recommended to take calcium and iron within 2 hours of each other.
5. Vitamin B12 can be taken orally, sublingually (under your tongue) and through intramuscular shots.
6. Oral vitamin B12 supplements are available in chewable form and dissolvable form.
7. Most over the counter vitamins are not suitable after bariatric surgery.
8. You need to take vitamins every day, for the rest of your life.
9. Women of child-bearing age need higher dosages of iron.

Chapter takeaways

- It can be challenging to meet your protein goals after bariatric surgery.
- The density of protein and feeling restricted in your meals, can contribute to this challenge.
- Breaking down your protein goal into smaller steps can be helpful to make the task less overwhelming.
- Keeping track of how much protein you're consuming, while also being aware of which foods contain protein, can help to meet your daily nutrition goals better.
- High-carbohydrate foods may not be the main focus right after surgery, but they do play an

important role in providing energy and offering a wide array of other nutrients in your diet.

- Knowing the difference between complex carbs and simple carbs can make all the difference in how you're utilizing this macronutrient after bariatric surgery.

- Alcohol is often not recommended within the first 12 months after bariatric surgery as it can increase the likelihood of dumping syndrome/digestive issues, takes away from other nutrition and health goals and possibly increases the risk of transfer addiction.

- Unsaturated fats help to get more vitamin A, D, E and K in. They also keep you more satisfied. Saturated fats on the other hand, should be limited.

- The micronutrient guidelines may differ depending on the bariatric surgery type. Mixed procedures like the gastric bypass or duodenal switch may require a higher dosage of post-operative supplements as the risk for malabsorption is higher as opposed to the gastric sleeve procedure for example.

- Working together with a dietitian, not only in the first year post-op, but also years later is helpful to make sure that you're meeting your nutritional goals better.

Chapter 7

7 Hydration tips that actually work

Dehydration is a serious risk for re-admittance within 30 days of having bariatric surgery. But even months down the line, you may still find yourself struggling to keep up with the daily hydration requirements. General guidelines state that after bariatric surgery a daily hydration intake of 64 ounces *(or nearly 2 liters)* is required. Your personal needs may differ of course, as variables like climate, physical exercise and certain medications that have a diuretic effect – may impact how many liquids you need.

To make sure that you're functioning properly and to help your digestive processes, hydration is a key element to successful nutrition post-op.

In this chapter we'll give you 7 tips to fall back on, whenever you feel like you can't keep up with your hydration goals. Let's get to it.

Why is it so hard to meet hydration goals after bariatric surgery?

Bariatric surgery should make you extra vigilant to stay on top of your hydration goals, as it becomes so much more challenging to keep up with a smaller stomach, changes in taste buds and a more sensitive digestive system.

If right now you're wondering, why it's so hard to meet your hydration goals after bariatric surgery, then let's break it down.

First of all, a smaller stomach means more restriction. This makes it more challenging to drink your liquids. On top of that, it's not recommended to gulp your liquids which makes the overall hydration process much slower and more tedious.

Another reason why bariatric surgery makes it harder to drink water specifically, is a possible change in taste buds. Water may leave a "metallic" taste in your mouth now that you had bariatric surgery.

And there's another pitfall when it comes down to staying hydrated.

After bariatric surgery, it's recommended to keep your solids separate from your liquids. This means that you have to get very intentional about timing your meals *and* drinks. Staying on top of your hydration goals, now becomes a full-time commitment.

So, how can you be more mindful about meeting your hydration goals? Here are 7 strategies to keep in mind.

Hydration Strategy #1 Break your hydration goal into smaller steps

If your goal is to drink 64 ounces of water daily, it may be helpful to break this number down in a way that makes sense *(just like we did with the protein goals, remember?)*. For example, if we break down the day into 4 quarters, your hydration goals could look something like this:

9:00 – 12:00 pm	**16 ounces**
12:00 – 3:00 pm	**16 ounces**
3:00 – 6:00 pm	**16 ounces**
6:00 – 9:00 pm	**16 ounces**

Customize this schedule to make it fitting to your own routine.

The point of this strategy is to make your overall goal feel less overwhelming. If you simply focus on the small steps in front of you, it's easier to get started and to keep going.

Hydration Strategy #2 Sipping around the clock

There should only be 3 reasons when you shouldn't be hydrating after bariatric surgery:

1. When you're eating.
2. When you're waiting after a meal to take your first sip.
3. When your schedule doesn't allow you to hydrate *(for example, you have a job that simply doesn't allow you to eat or drink while working)*.

Taking small sips in between your meals and chores, is a simple but effective strategy to get more liquids in.

Hydration Strategy #3 Rehydration after the restroom

You're using the restroom multiple times a day. So, why not make it a habit to hydrate after using the restroom? Use the sequence: "pee" → "hydrate" and turn it into an automated process if you're struggling with staying hydrated.

By checking the color and smell of your urine, you can gauge if you need more liquids or not.

Is your urine too dark *(dark-yellow, (light) orange)*? Then this is your visual sign to drink more water. Is your urine particularly strong-smelling? Then this is your olfactory sign to drink more water.

Signs that could implicate dehydration are: dizziness, foggy brain, dry mouth and throat, headaches, muscle cramps and fatigue.

Hydration Strategy #4 Keep track to create awareness

If you're busy, not thirsty or simply forgetful, it's easier to stray from your hydration goals. Here's where tracking how much liquids you had in a day, can be incredibly helpful to get those ounces *(or liters)* in.

Try using a simple hydration tracker, so that you can keep a close eye on your liquids *(there's one included in the freebies at the beginning of this book!)*.

Hydration Strategy #5 Tackle water nausea

When we talk about hydration, the number one liquid we think of is water. But bariatric surgery can dramatically change your experience with drinking water. As mentioned before, water may taste different, leaving a somewhat metallic taste in your mouth. Or perhaps drinking water makes you nauseous, making it seem impossible to meet the requirements.

If regular water is hard to tolerate, then these strategies should be taken into consideration *(all in consultation with your care team of course)*:

- Natural flavor enhancers, like mint or ginger.
- Herbal teas, like peppermint or chamomile tea.
- Water with electrolytes.
- Alkaline water.
- Sugar-free flavor enhancer packets.
- Straws *(only if they don't cause any gas, bloating or discomfort)*.
- Different brands mineral water; sometimes having a different ratio of minerals can be helpful.
- Ice chips and ice cubes made from plain water.

How long does water nausea persist? There's no clear-cut

answer. Perhaps your symptoms are only temporary, or maybe you still can't tolerate water years later.

Hydration Strategy #6 Experiment with temperature

You may find yourself tolerating warm drinks better than cold ones. Or the other way around.
Try adding ice cubes to your water and see if that helps. Maybe some warm tea will do the trick. Or perhaps serving your drink at room temperature is just what your stomach needs.
Keep in mind that ice-cold, or very hot beverages are not recommended right after surgery when your stomach is still healing.

Hydration Strategy #7 Eat foods high in water

Although foods high in water don't count towards your total hydration goals, it sure helps to quench the thirst. Here are a few examples of foods that also have a high-water content:

- Watermelon
- Cantaloupe
- Cucumber
- Zucchini
- Lettuce
- Strawberries
- Blueberries
- Tomatoes

- Broccoli

Straws after bariatric surgery

So, can you or can't you use straws after bariatric surgery? There doesn't seem to be any scientific research that states that straws can expand your stomach. However, using a straw could lead into taking larger sips, which could possibly lead to more swallowing of air. And this may cause bloating or discomfort.

But the upside of using a straw after bariatric surgery, is that for many, it becomes easier to meet daily hydration goals.

Our best tip? Ask your surgeon what's best for you. And also, don't forget to ask *"why, is that?"*. Learn how to lean into your own body's cues, as you may quickly learn what feels right and what doesn't.

There's no right or wrong when it comes down to this topic, but only what is right for you within your own context. If drinking through a straw doesn't cause any discomfort, but it helps you hit your hydration goals compared to when you don't use one – then using a straw seems nothing more than common sense.

But if using a straw result in pain, bloating or discomfort – then obviously it's better to refrain from using one. Especially when you just had bariatric surgery.

Carbonation after bariatric surgery

Most surgeons will recommend <u>not</u> to use any carbonated beverages after bariatric surgery. There doesn't seem to be any experimental research indicating that carbonation can cause pouch stretching. But they do seem to have other downsides to keep in mind:

- Carbonated beverages may increase the risk of acid reflux.
- Sodas may contain too many added sugars which goes against the guideline to minimize added sugars after bariatric surgery.
- Drinking soda may also trigger old eating habits that weren't helpful.
- Carbonated beverages may cause pain, bloating and discomfort.
- Carbonated beverages may make you full quicker, which could take away from meeting other nutritional goals *(if you're full, it's less likely you will eat a nutritious meal)*.

Coffee and other caffeinated beverages after bariatric surgery

What about drinking coffee? What are the consequences of caffeine if you had weight loss surgery? Most surgeons will agree that caffeine should be avoided in the early stages after bariatric surgery. A 30-day time frame seems acceptable, but if and when you should add caffeine to your daily routine should be discussed with your surgeon.

Caffeine is NOT recommended during the recovery period for 2 main reasons:

1. Although the notion that caffeine leads to dehydration, seems to be less supported nowadays. It's important to remain cautious.
2. Caffeine can be an irritant to the lining of your stomach. When you had surgery, your stomach is still healing. Anything that may cause irritation, should be avoided.

Once you're cleared to have coffee again, there are ways to make your coffee more nutritious. This can be done by making a so-called "proffee". A beverage where a high-protein milk product and coffee are combined.

What about alcohol?
In Chapter 6 we discussed all the details about alcohol use after bariatric surgery. Go back to page 67 to refresh your memory.

Chapter takeaways

- Not drinking together with your meals, high restriction and not being able to gulp, makes it more challenging to meet hydration goals.
- Bariatric friendly alternatives to water and drinking your water at a different serving temperature are strategies that can help you meet your hydration goals better.
- There seems to be no scientific evidence that straws or carbonation could lead to stomach stretching.

- However, the use of straws could lead to bloating and discomfort. On the other hand, using straws could also make it easier to hit hydration goals.
- The use of carbonated beverages is usually advised against as this could increase the risk of acid reflux, pain, bloating and discomfort. Also, carbonated beverages in the form of soda are advised against because of their high-sugar properties.

Chapter 8

How to preserve muscle mass (and why it's important to do so)

Not all weight loss is the same. In this chapter we show you the importance of muscle mass and we give you 3 tips to preserve more muscles once you had bariatric surgery.

This is why muscle mass matters

Here are the facts.

Bariatric surgery puts you at a higher risk of losing muscles. The most common reason is the daily challenge to eat enough protein, combined with insufficient physical activity to promote muscle maintenance or growth.

When your stomach is reduced and your hunger hormones decrease, it's a strenuous task to get enough nutrients in. Especially when your restriction is high.

But why is it so important to maintain your muscle mass? Let's explain.

Muscle mass is an indicator of overall health. When your muscles deteriorate, your immune system weakens. You lose your strength and it's more likely that your hair and nails suffer too.

Your muscle mass is partly responsible for the rate of your metabolism. We call this the *basal metabolic rate (BMR)*: the minimum energy required to perform basic functions in your body to stay alive. For example, your heart beat, digestive processes and breathing.

If you lose muscles, your metabolic rate slows down. And a slower BMR is associated with poorer weight loss outcomes. Simply put: you need muscle mass to lose weight. In particular, fat tissue.

Now, let's look at 3 things you can focus on, to make sure that you keep muscle loss to a minimum.

#1 Protein is the key macronutrient

Fun fact: your body doesn't have the ability to store protein. This means you need a daily dose of protein to maintain your muscles *(remember: protein is THE building block of your muscles)*.

But it's not just protein that help you retain your muscular tissue. Studies suggest that adding a small amount of (complex) carbs to your protein-packed meal, helps to build more muscles quicker. And this is how that works:

When eating carbohydrates, your body breaks this down into glucose. Glucose is your energy source for your cells. When glucose hits the blood stream, insulin production is activated so that glucose can be transported to your cells for energy. Insulin is an *anabolic hormone.* In other words: it builds. And what it also does, it aids in muscle repair and muscle maintenance too.

#2 Use your muscles to fuel your muscles

There's two ways to preserve your muscles. One is through a high-protein diet, and the second way is through exercise. Light resistance training can be helpful to keep muscle loss to a minimum.

Make sure to follow your surgeon's guidelines when it comes down to incorporating exercise again.

#3 Stop skipping meals and cease the opportunity

When you skip your meals, you also turn down an opportunity to eat protein. This takes away from your daily protein goal. If you skimp on the number of meals you're having in a day, you're missing out on pivotal moments to get your protein in.

"But how many times should I eat?"

This depends on the following:

- How much protein are you able to eat in one sitting? If you can only manage 10g of protein per meal, then you'd have to eat a minimum of 6 times a day to get the minimum requirement of 60g of protein in.

- How are you feeling? If you feel dizzy, unsatiated or need more energy from food – then eating 3 times a day may not be enough. Incorporating snacks in between your meals can be a great way of feeling better.

- What is a realistic eating schedule for you? For example, if you're working long shifts without any breaks – it becomes so much more challenging to add those "eating moments" into your waking hours. Personal advice is recommended to make sure you do hit your nutrition goals, while also feeling energized.

Chapter takeaways

- Bariatric surgery puts you at a greater risk of losing muscle mass.
- Muscle loss is associated with loss of strength, longer post-op recovery times, slower weight loss and weight regain.
- Focusing on protein and exercise are ways to minimize muscle loss.
- Working with a dietitian can give you more insight about which nutrition-strategies work best for your personal lifestyle.

Part 3

The best strategies for top-notch eating habits

Chapter 9

Understanding appetite and restriction

Changing your eating habits is hard. And one of the reasons, is that physical hunger is complex in light of obesity. Also, bariatric surgery may initially reduce physical hunger, but its effects aren't ever-lasting. Appetite does return, which is normal, but it can feel intimidating if you can't fully grasp why that is. To fully breakdown the concept of appetite and restriction we have to discuss a few key elements, which are:

- Hormones that drive appetite and satiety: ghrelin and leptin
- Other factors that impact hunger: sleep deprivation and stress
- Mind hunger and emotional eating
- Restriction after bariatric surgery

Ghrelin: the hunger hormone

Ghrelin is a hormone that's mainly produced in the upper part of the stomach *(the fundus)* and was discovered in 1999. Ghrelin is called the "hunger hormone" because it increases appetite and initiates eating. Ghrelin levels rise before having a meal and they drop after finishing a meal.

Before bariatric surgery, you had more ghrelin receptors than after bariatric surgery. After any type of bariatric procedure, either a majority of the ghrelin production sites are removed *(after a sleeve for example)*, or bypassed *(like in the gastric bypass)*. This simple anatomical change is one of the reasons for a decrease in appetite. On top of that, bariatric surgery improves sensitivity to ghrelin, restoring the balance of hunger hormone regulation.

Leptin: the satiety hormone

Leptin is produced in your fat cells and was discovered in 1994. Leptin is also known as the "fullness" or "satiety" hormone as it signals your brain that you're full. The more body fat you have, the more leptin you produce. Now, you would expect that the more leptin, the quicker you feel full, right? But unfortunately, this is not the case.

You see, obesity causes *leptin resistance*. And when you're leptin resistant, your body becomes insensitive to leptin, making it lose its purpose of letting you know that you're full.

Imagine your experience with eating before bariatric surgery. Perhaps you can relate to a constant nagging feeling of hunger and not getting the signal that you're feeling full. Maybe you did get this signal, but it always came too late. This is a sign that your hunger hormones were out of balance, making it so much harder not to "give in" to the urge to eat. On top of that, it's also more challenging to stop eating if you don't feel satiated. Obesity is truly a metabolic illness and that's why a lack of sheer willpower is NOT a great argument in the light of losing weight and obesity.

After bariatric surgery, you lose weight. As you're losing weight, a part of your fat mass also decreases which means that your leptin levels drop. But most importantly, your body becomes more sensitive to leptin again. Your feelings of fullness have returned and are much more noticeable after bariatric surgery!

As you're connecting with your new hunger and satiety cues after bariatric surgery, it becomes easier to stop when you're actually feeling full.

Keep in mind that hunger and satiety are experienced differently by everyone. It's common to experience hunger shortly after bariatric surgery and it's also common to not feel hungry even months later down the line. You could be someone who is fine-tuned with your fullness cues, knowing exactly when it's time to stop eating. Or perhaps you still have a hard time gauging when you're full.

Practicing mindful eating, helps to become more aware of all of your eating cues, both before and after bariatric surgery.

Other factors that impact hunger: sleep and stress

Sleep and appetite
A good night's sleep is not only valuable because you feel better when well-rested, it's also helpful in managing your

hunger cues. Research shows that sleep deprivation can lead to an:

- Increased calorie intake
- Increased "hedonic effect" of food *(food becomes more appealing)*

When you're tired, you lack energy. And it's common sense that you may start looking for energy in food to compensate for your fatigue. On top of that, some foods that already have a greater effect on the pleasure and reward center of the brain *(like high-sugar foods or fried foods)*, are amplified by sleep deprivation. When you're tired, a piece of chocolate can become more appealing than when you had a good night's rest.

If you had bariatric surgery, it's important to be aware of how sleep can impact the food choices you make the next day.

Stress and appetite

According to the Oxford dictionary, stress is a *"state of mental or emotion strain or tension resulting from adverse or demanding circumstances"*.

Stress can stem from many different life circumstances and events. Stress is also subjective: what may be stressful for one person isn't stressful for somebody else. The key point is, that stress often takes a greater toll on overall health than you may realize.

The hormone that increases when we're feeling stressed is *cortisol*. Cortisol puts your body in a "flight-or-fight" mode, increasing your carbohydrate and fat metabolism which leads to a sudden surge of energy in your body. This is a helpful response when there's actual danger and we need to take action.

The issue with most stressors nowadays, is that they are chronic. They last for too long and even if the stressor is long gone, your body may have gotten used to this constant feeling of stress.

Not only does stress have many negative implications for overall health, it also results in a greater appetite. Not surprisingly, cortisol doesn't lead to an appetite in whole nutritious foods, but cause cravings for sweet, salty or fatty foods; high-caloric foods that give quick energy.

Living entirely stress-free is unrealistic, but when you're chronically stressed, your health goals after bariatric surgery are also compromised.

How to decompress and minimize stress? Here are just a handful of examples to take into consideration:

- Journaling
- Talking about your feelings with someone you trust
- Physical exercise
- Meditating
- Praying
- Breathing exercises
- Acceptance of the things you *can't* control
- Problem solving for the things you *can* control
- Setting boundaries

Mind hunger and emotional eating

So far, we discussed some of the mechanisms that drive physical hunger: ghrelin, leptin, sleep deprivation and stress (cortisol).

But what about emotional eating? How can you tackle mind hunger after bariatric surgery?

Emotional eating can be defined as eating in response to emotions. Emotional eating is a coping mechanism to distract yourself from feeling the overwhelm stemming from certain emotions. Food may have always been a safe resort dating back to childhood, when you felt emotionally unsafe. Food may have become a coping mechanism because the obstacles in your life, were too immense to deal with. Perhaps you didn't have any other tools when it came down to dealing with major life stress events, trauma or other difficulties that were thrown your way.

If you've never learned how to navigate your feelings, without the self-blame, self-loathing and judgment you may feel, it's going to be challenging to overcome emotional eating.

Bariatric surgery doesn't automatically "fix" any underlying causes for a disrupted relationship with food. So, not surprisingly, it doesn't do much for emotional eating either. However, bariatric surgery can create more awareness as you may notice not to be able to eat the foods your brain craves.

Emotional eating, mind hunger, emotional cravings – they all boil down to the same thing. Coping with feelings through food.

So, in order to face emotional eating, it's invaluable to work on your *emotional well-being*. It's key to find new coping mechanism to work through the feelings that may seem too overwhelming to deal with.

Journaling, (cognitive-behavioral) therapy and meditation are just a handful of means to work *with* your emotions instead of suppressing them.

Because the harsh truth is this: if you don't work on healing your relationship with food, bariatric surgery won't do the healing for you.

Bariatric surgery forces you to take on a whole new way of eating, making emotional cravings and mind hunger perhaps even more apparent. If food aversions, a smaller stomach and a decreased physical appetite block the ability to use food as a coping mechanism – then the emotional strain that has been suppressed before, becomes more tangible.

On the other hand, if you're further out of surgery and notice that your eating pattern becomes more normalized in the sense that you can tolerate most foods and you don't feel your restriction as much as you did in the beginning – certain foods *(slider foods)* can become a true pitfall if you stop working on your (emotional) eating habits.

Rome wasn't built overnight. Healing your relationship with food may take longer than your 1-year Surgiversary. And that's okay. Being a work in progress is never something to be sad or ashamed about. Personal growth should be praised and you have to come to terms that your bariatric journey extends way beyond the honeymoon stage.

And for the record, emotional eating in moderation, is completely healthy human behavior. Emotions are part life, and it's nothing out of the ordinary if you eat cake because it's your birthday and you're happy. It's also normal to crave chocolate when you're feeling down, for example. Where it becomes tricky is the number of times this happens and the amount of trigger foods you allow in your diet. It becomes an issue when you don't have any other coping mechanisms or strategies to deal with life's adversities.

Restriction: why does it fluctuate after bariatric surgery?

Have you ever noticed that one day you can eat a full plate of solid food, while the next, you can barely eat a spoonful of food, because you're too full?

No matter what bariatric surgery procedure you had, the size of your stomach is drastically reduced. In other words: bariatric surgery causes *restriction* due to reducing the size of your stomach's capacity to hold a meal.

The feeling of restriction is subjective, meaning that everyone experiences their restriction, and thus the amount of food consumed in one sitting, differently.

We refer to high restriction when you feel full quickly. And we refer to low restriction when you don't feel full quickly. Now, "quickly" is an entirely subjective term once again. But you probably know first-hand what we mean. On some days your stomach feels like a bottomless pit, while on others – you feel stuffed all day long.

Now, let's look at one of the first reasons why restriction changes over time: the healing of your pouch.

The natural decline of your restriction: time after surgery

This one isn't rocket-science. The simple fact that time passes, causes your restriction to slowly decrease *(in time, it's normal that appetite kicks back in)*.

And there's two physical reasons for that:

- Your pouch is healing after surgery
- Your hunger hormones are likely to rise in time

What really happens when the swelling in your stomach subsides

After bariatric surgery your stomach is still swollen. Your surgeon puts you on a post-op diet and the road to recovery has begun. Not only does the smaller size of your new stomach causes restriction, the swelling plays a part too.

Once the swelling subsides, you notice that you're able to eat more. This is in line with your post-op diet where you gradually add more foods and textures to your diet.

Now let's move on to the next reason for your restriction to fluctuate: the way you're eating.

Mindful eating and the link to your restriction

Mindful eating refers to being fully present and aware when you're consuming a meal. And it could imply the following:

- Thinking about the food you're eating while you eat
- Savoring the taste and texture of your food
- Eating slow and chewing well

The latter is especially relevant when we're talking about your restriction. You see, it takes about 20 minutes for your stomach to signal your brain that you're approaching fullness. If you're eating too fast, you may miss that fullness cue completely – ignoring your restriction.

Three questions to ask yourself when you're trying to make sense of your restriction after bariatric surgery

So far, we discussed time out of surgery and the pace of your eating as predictors of your fluctuating restriction.

Now let's move on to 3 questions you can ask yourself whenever you restriction feels different all of the sudden.

1. "What did I eat that caused my restriction to feel different?"

What you eat has an effect on your restriction. But how does that work exactly?

Let's get to the bottom of it.

If you eat meals that are high in protein, fiber and healthy fats, you're maximizing your restriction. Protein, fiber and unsaturated fats promote a healthy way of satiety. In other words: these nutrients keep you full for longer. Also, high-protein meals lead to a drop in ghrelin levels making you feel less hungry too.

But if you're eating slider foods, your restriction decreases. Slider foods tend to slide through your stomach much faster as they become liquid quick and take little time to digest. This leaves you unsatisfied and hungrier quicker. Simply put: your restriction is less noticeable when you eat slider foods. More about slider foods in Chapter 12.

2. "Did my restriction change because I was physically active?"

If you've been working out more, or increased your daily movement, it's more likely that your appetite increased as well. This is the simple consequence of needing more energy, as your metabolism increased.

As a result of more appetite, usually, less restriction follows naturally.

3. "Am I stressed? Did this affect my restriction?"

As we discussed in the previous section, stress can have a great impact on your eating habits. If you're stressed, it could lead to less restriction as your appetite may have increased.

On the other hand, some people may feel like they "shut down" making it hard to eat anything when stressed.

Chapter takeaways

- Hunger and satiety hormones like ghrelin and leptin drive appetite.
- Bariatric surgery sensitizes these mechanisms leading to a re-balance of the hunger-satiety-mechanisms.
- Stress and sleep deprivation can negatively impact food choices and weight loss outcomes.
- Restriction is the subjective feeling of "fullness" and differs across situations and individuals.

Chapter 10

How to prevent overeating

Overeating with a small stomach? It may sound counter-intuitive, but overeating after bariatric surgery is not impossible. Especially when you're further out of surgery and you notice you're able to tolerate a wider variety of foods and your portions naturally increase.

When overeating becomes a pattern you may risk:

- Weight regain
- Pouch stretching
- Opening the floodgates for disruptive eating habits

In this chapter we give you simple tips on how to prevent overeating as much as you possibly can.

The mechanisms behind appetite: restriction and hunger hormones

As we discussed in the previous chapter, physical hunger is mainly driven by hormones such as ghrelin and leptin. The likelihood of overeating is greater when you constantly have an urge to eat and/or when you can't tell when you're approaching fullness. After bariatric surgery, both sensitivity to ghrelin and leptin improves.

However, if new eating habits aren't sustained long term, ghrelin and leptin can become imbalanced again. It's important to be aware of the mechanisms that drive physical hunger and how they change after bariatric surgery. Now, let's move on to the two types of overeating that can occur.

Types of overeating explained

We can make a distinction between two different ways of overeating:

1. Overeating during one meal sitting
Now, overeating in "one go" typically happens when you eat too fast or aren't paying attention to your *fullness cues.*

2. Overeating throughout the entire day
If you're overeating throughout the day, you may find yourself grazing.

"Grazing is defined as unplanned eating and nibbling away mindlessly on small amounts of (slider) foods over a longer period of time".

Grazing can happen when you're not able to finish a proper solid meal, feeling full too quickly – but yet hungry within minutes after your last bite. It feels like you constantly need to eat to hit your goals and to stay nourished.

Or perhaps the cause of grazing is *emotional eating,* making it harder to stop eating, despite the lack of an appetite.

How to prevent overeating after bariatric surgery

Now that we explained what overeating is, let's look at different strategies to prevent overeating, or at least, be more mindful about it.

1. Pay attention to your fullness cues

As we discussed in the previous chapter, the way you experience hunger and fullness changes tremendously once you had bariatric surgery. And to refresh your memory, here are 6 fullness-cues to look out for:

- Burping
- Hiccups
- Yawning
- Sneezing
- Coughing
- Runny nose

2. Eat slow and chew well to prevent overeating

It takes about 20 minutes for your brain to let your stomach know that you're full. Eating slow helps to recognize your fullness cues in time. More strategies to eat slower are presented in Chapter 13.

3. Add protein and fiber to your meals and snacks

Both protein and fiber are invaluable nutrients after bariatric surgery. Besides needing protein and fiber for numerous health reasons, like muscle preservation and gut health – protein and fiber are filling. And thus help to curb appetite, because they maximize your restriction. Also, healthy fats found in most nuts and seeds, avocado, fatty fish and plant-based oils – create satiety while also providing you a wide array of nutrients and fat-soluble vitamins, such as vitamin A, D, E and K.

4. Avoid drinking together with your meals

Why can't you drink together with your meals? What happens when you do that?

Well, when you drink together with your meals you "flush" down your foods more easily through your stomach. Which in turn leads to an empty stomach, faster. This in turn increases the risk of overeating.

On top of that, drinking together with your meals can trigger dumping syndrome. A very unpleasant side-effect after bariatric surgery that can completely catch you off guard *(we'll discuss the details of dumping syndrome in the next chapter)*.

Generally, it's recommended to wait 30 minutes after eating before you take your first sip. And some surgeons may even advice to also wait 30 minutes after drinking to take your first bite. That means you're on a very tight eating and drinking schedule if you want to make sure to get all your nutrients and liquids in.

5. Put your food on a plate

It's easier to overeat when you "snack" out of the bag or package, then when you
put your food on a plate or in a bowl. The visualization of your meal as a whole, helps to stimulate your fullness cues.

6. Small plate, small utensils

Visuals can make a huge difference in your eating habits after bariatric surgery. If your food intake is decreased, but you're still using regular plates and utensils – it may look like you're eating "too little". And this can be confusing.

By using smaller plates *(8-9 inches or 20-22 centimeters)* and smaller utensils, it becomes visually more appealing to eat a smaller amount of food. It also helps to slow down your eating pace when your bites are smaller too.

7. Single serve packets

Portion control matters. And if you're buying pre-packed foods, the serving size can play a role in how much you feel like you "should" be eating. If you're used to finishing your plate or eating the entire serving, then having smaller serve packets can be helpful to prevent overeating.

Foods that may come in smaller single serve packets are:

- Nuts and seeds
- String cheese

- Protein chips
- Fruit packets
- Veggie packets
- Yogurts
- Protein puddings

Chapter takeaways

- Overeating on a consistent basis can lead to complications such as weight regain or stomach stretching.
- Overeating can be prevented by using strategies, such as eating slow, being aware of fullness cues, separating solids from liquids and creating visually appealing plates that help with portion control.

Chapter 11

How to prevent dumping syndrome

Up to 70% of bariatric surgery patients experience dumping syndrome at least once after their surgery. But not all dumping syndrome is the same. What exactly is dumping syndrome? And are there ways to prevent it from happening? We shed more light on this unpleasant side-effect in this chapter.

What is dumping syndrome?

To answer this question, we first need to make a distinction between early dumping syndrome and late dumping syndrome.

Early dumping syndrome
As the name already applies, early dumping syndrome occurs quickly after eating, about 10-30 minutes after a meal. And early dumping symptoms may include:

- Bloating
- Diarrhea
- Nausea
- Lightheadedness
- Sweating
- Vomiting

- Heart palpitations
- Rapid heart rate

And what happens anatomically is this:

Undigested, calorie-dense liquids or solids trigger something called *hyperosmolarity* in the inside of your intestines *(the lumen)*, leading to fluids being drawn *into* your small intestine. The higher the osmolarity in the lumen, the more fluid is drawn towards it.

Let's explain a bit more.

Hypertonic liquids are liquids with a higher concentrated level of sugars such as juice. These types of drinks trigger dumping syndrome more easily through the process of osmosis. The result might be diarrhea.

The most common triggers for early dumping syndrome are:

- Eating or drinking foods high in refined carbs *(for example, cookies, ice cream and milkshakes)*
- Eating or drinking foods high in fats
- Drinking together with your meals

If you experience early dumping, you may find that lying down can somewhat relief the symptoms.

Late dumping syndrome
Late dumping syndrome is also known as *reactive hypoglycemia* or *postprandial dumping syndrome* and is triggered

by an exaggerated insulin response. Symptoms of late dumping syndrome may look like this:

- Anxiety
- Sweating
- Heart palpitations
- Weakness
- Strong sugar cravings
- Fatigue
- Fainting
- Diarrhea
- Rapid heart rate
- Confusion
- Problems concentrating

If you're suffering from late dumping syndrome, you may find that these things can help:

- Eating a reasonable amount of sugar to normalize blood sugar levels again. It could be as simple as a glucose tab. Always find out what works best for you.
- Lying down, especially if you feel faint or dizzy.
- Monitoring your blood glucose levels to get a better understanding of how your body responds to certain foods.
- Keeping a food journal to get more perspective about your so-called trigger foods.

How to minimize dumping syndrome

You can't always prevent dumping syndrome, even if you're very mindful about what you eat and the way you eat. But here are 4 strategies to keep in mind when trying to keep dumping syndrome at bay:

Avoid refined sugars and foods that have a high glycemic index

Examples of refined sugars are white sugar, brown sugar and high-fructose corn syrup. These sugars have been processed to keep their sweet taste as much as possible when incorporated into different food sources. Refined sugars have a higher glycemic index and are digested much quicker than complex carbs for example. The higher the glycemic index, the quicker the food raises your blood sugar levels.

After bariatric surgery, it's important to be mindful of refined sugars in the foods and drinks you consume as they can trigger dumping syndrome much quicker. And to make things even more complicated, sugar isn't always labeled as "sugar" on a food label. There are tons of different ingredients that fall into the "sugar category". The list below includes both refined sugars and sugars that are naturally found in foods:

1. Sucrose
2. High fructose corn syrup (HFCS)
3. Dextrose
4. Glucose
5. Fructose
6. Maltose

7. Lactose
8. Galactose
9. Brown sugar
10. Molasses
11. Cane sugar
12. Invert sugar
13. Raw sugar
14. Turbinado sugar
15. Confectioner's sugar
16. Evaporated cane juice
17. Fruit juice concentrate
18. Corn syrup
19. Agave nectar
20. Honey
21. Maple syrup
22. Rice syrup
23. Barley malt
24. Coconut sugar
25. Date sugar

But it's not just sugar that causes dumping syndrome. Bariatric patients also report a variety of other food characteristics *(like, food that is too fat or too spicy)* that led to a dumping episode.

You see, the quicker food passes from your stomach to your small intestine, the more likely you experience dumping syndrome. What you want to aim for after bariatric surgery, is a slower transit from food from your stomach to the rest of your digestive system.

So, how can you slow down this transit? Well, separating your solids from your liquids is the next strategy to keep in mind.

Separate your solid food from your liquids

Adding liquids to solids makes your food more liquid. And this in turn leads to faster *gastric emptying*. In other words, your food passes through from stomach to your small intestine more quickly. And as mentioned above, a quicker transit trough your small intestine increases the risk for dumping syndrome. By separating your solid food from your beverages, you allow more time between the emptying of your stomach and the passage of food in your small intestine.

Eat slow and chew well

When you swallow your food too fast, the quicker that food is deployed (or "dumped") in your small intestine. Chewing well allows more time to digest your food better and thus reducing the risk of dumping syndrome.

Tune into your body's cues

What causes dumping syndrome for one person, may not cause the same symptoms for somebody else. ***Lean into your own body's cues.*** Once you start to eat more mindfully, you get more acquainted with your new stomach. For example, some people experience more frequent dumping syndrome episodes when consuming foods high in lactose. A lactose-free diet may be beneficial for those who became sensitive to lactose after bariatric surgery.

But keep in mind that even if you didn't experience digestive issues with a type of food one day, that doesn't mean that you can't experience digestive issues with the same food another day. Simply put: dumping syndrome is not always predictable and can really catch you by surprise.

Chapter takeaways

- Dumping syndrome is an unpleasant side-effect after bariatric surgery.
- Foods that are high in added sugars are most likely to trigger dumping syndrome.
- But any type of food or way of eating that evokes a quicker transit from stomach to the small intestine, can cause dumping syndrome.
- Early dumping occurs quickly after eating and the symptoms include nausea, diarrhea and vomiting.
- Reactive hypoglycemia, or late dumping syndrome, is an exaggerated insulin response causing hypoglycemic symptoms like feeling faint and dizzy.
- Keeping track of your food triggers and leaning into your new body's cues is helpful to understand your physical responses to food better after bariatric surgery.

Chapter 12

The truth about slider foods

By now, we've mentioned slider foods more than once. And now it's time to really get into the details of what slider foods are and why it's important to be mindful about them after bariatric surgery.

What are slider foods?

Slider foods are high-carbohydrate foods that are low in protein and/or have little fiber. And if you remembered well, you now know that carbohydrate digestion starts in your mouth with an enzyme called *amylase*. This means, that part of the slider food is already digested before it enters the stomach. Slider foods by themselves, result in a quicker transit from stomach to small intestine. And they tend to have the following characteristics:

- They don't keep you full for long
- They need little time to digest
- They're low in nutritional value *(high in sugar, but low in protein, fiber, unsaturated fats, vitamins and minerals)*
- It's easy to overeat or overindulge in them
- They're often trigger foods too

Now, we're not going to label slider foods as "bad" foods. But it is important to be mindful of all slider foods as they can sabotage weight loss after bariatric surgery. On top of that, slider foods can become a pitfall for disrupted eating patterns.

List of slider foods

Keep in mind that the list below is very generic. If we talk about "cookies" there's tons of different types and variations. Some cookies may have more protein and fiber than others.

But to give you a general idea, here's what type of foods to look out for:

- Chips
- Nachos
- Pretzels
- Crackers
- Cookies
- Chocolate
- Candy
- Milkshakes
- Cake
- Popcorn
- Ice cream

How to navigate slider foods after bariatric surgery

Again, slider foods aren't bad foods, but they're not the type of foods that are going to help you meet your post-op nutritional goals when eaten on a daily basis, in larger quantities. And because they become liquid quickly and digest faster, it's so much easier to overeat on slider foods. You may find it easier to eat a few cookies than a hard-boiled egg. The slider food is not nutrient dense, while the egg is. Being aware of the nutrient density of different foods, helps to understand why you're able to eat more of one food than the other.

When slider foods are eaten by themselves, it can be tempting to consume larger quantities. It may seem like you've stretched your stomach, but in reality, it's just easier to eat more slider foods than nutrient-dense foods.

When eating slider foods, you might:

1. Sabotage weight loss because of their high-caloric characteristics
2. Risk dumping syndrome because of their high-sugar characteristics

So, is there something you can do to create balance on your plate? Is it possible to enjoy some slider foods in moderation when you're further out of surgery, so that you're not falling for an *all-or-nothing mentality*, later down the line?

Actually, there is a way to be mindful without restricting yourself for the rest of your life.

By adding high-protein, high-fiber foods and foods that contain unsaturated fats, you create balance. In other words: if you add *nutritious foods* to your meals and snacks, you honor your hunger – and you minimize cravings too.

And here are a handful of examples:

- Cheese *(e.g., cheese paired with crackers)*
- Any type of dairy product, like Greek yogurt *(e.g., chips paired with a Greek yogurt dip)*
- Legumes *(e.g., nachos paired with a hummus dip)*
- Fruit *(e.g., grapes paired with popcorn)*
- Vegetables *(e.g., deli plate with carrots, cucumber and crackers)*

Chapter takeaways

- Slider foods aren't necessarily "bad" *(remember, we don't demonize foods, but we do need to be mindful about which foods serve your purpose and which ones don't).*
- Slider foods can negatively impact your weight loss journey.
- Slider foods can be a pitfall for disruptive eating patterns as they're often also trigger foods that immediately affect the reward center in the brain.
- Slider foods are low in nutritional value but have a high hedonic effect *(they look appealing).*
- Slider foods, when eaten by themselves, won't keep you full for long.
- Pairing slider foods with protein, fiber and/or unsaturated fat, makes your snack more filling and nutritious.

Chapter 13

4 Simple tips to eat slower

What you eat after bariatric surgery is important. But *how* you eat, matters too.

Eating slow sounds simple. But this is far from true. The process of eating, chewing and swallowing is mostly automated. This means that it becomes so much more challenging to be mindful about it. You hardly ever have to think about chewing and swallowing your food, because your subconscious already has that part covered.

But after bariatric surgery, your digestive system changes dramatically. You're forced to practice new eating habits, because otherwise you risk digestive issues, discomfort or pain. Hence, eating slow is one of the bariatric basics to always keep in mind.

In this chapter we give you 4 simple tips to eat slower. But first, let's learn more why it's necessary to pace yourself.

Why is it important to eat slow after bariatric surgery?

You may wonder why it's recommended to eat slower once you had bariatric surgery. Well, there are 2 main reasons we'd like to point out.

First, if you eat too fast, you're more likely to overeat. As mentioned before, it takes about 20 minutes for your stomach to signal your brain that you're full. If you eat too fast, you miss this cue.

Second, eating fast can cause digestive issues. Bariatric surgery changes the digestive system which automatically puts you at higher risk for digestive complications like nausea, stomach pain and vomiting. Eating fast can amplify these symptoms.

It's usually recommended to chew at least 20 times on each bite before you swallow. For some foods this makes more sense than for others. Chewing on a raspberry is completely different than chewing on a piece of steak. A bite of yogurt barely requires any chewing at all. You can always fall back on the rule of thumb that your food should have the texture of apple sauce before you swallow: soft, mushy and chunk-free.

Now let's move on to our 4 best tips to slow down when eating:

1. Push your plate away after each bite

This strategy makes most sense when at home. Shifting your plate back and forth in social settings can be awkward, and that's more than understandable. The "pushing plate" method will slow down your eating process and could help to recognize your fullness cues quicker.

2. Put down your utensils after each bite

It may feel unnatural to keep putting down and picking up your utensils while you're eating. But there's 2 reasons why this technique can help you slow down:

- You're more mindful of the pace of your eating by just setting the intention to do this
- It takes more time to finish your meal this way

3. Do what *you* need to slow down: say yes to distractions or say no to distractions

It truly depends on how your digestive system responds when you're eating. When you just had bariatric surgery and you're still introducing new foods and textures to your diet, you may find yourself chewing on each bite meticulously before swallowing *(while anticipating anxiously whether that bite will get stuck or not)*.

4. Don't put food in your mouth when there's food in your mouth

Make sure to swallow every bite before you take another one. Don't take a bite when you're still chewing.

But things might change.

Once you're further out and you discover that you don't have to eat that "carefully" any longer *(at least not to prevent digestive issues)*, you may find yourself eating in a hurry again.

But we're here to emphasize that slowing down remains important throughout your journey.

If turning off the television, phone or tablet works for you – then do that. But if you find yourself eating more slowly when you are "distracted" by other things – then that may be a better strategy for you.

Slow, but not too slow

Eating slow is important, but there's a caveat. *Too slow* isn't always better. When it takes you longer than 30 minutes to finish one meal, it's time to stop eating. The reason behind this, is that eating too slow promotes grazing behavior. And grazing is one of the main reasons for weight regain after bariatric surgery.

Also, if you continue to eat for more than 30 minutes per meal, you probably miss your fullness cues quicker, because you may not feel satiated. If you want to aim for the right timing, set a 20–25-minute to set the right pace.

Chapter takeaways

- Eating slow helps to prevent digestive issues.
- When you slow down, you notice your fullness cues in time. This in turn helps to prevent overeating.
- The sweet spot to finish a meal is around 20 minutes. But this is dependent on what type of meal you're having and if the food itself requires lots of chewing or not. Not all meals require 20 minutes to finish. Make sure that you set realistic

goals for yourself without losing sight of the basic guidelines.

Part 4

Hold on to a brand-new mindset

Chapter 14

How to stop the scale from dictating your mood

The scale. Let's talk about it.

It goes without saying that weight loss is an important part of bariatric surgery. Especially during the honeymoon stage *(12-18 months post-op)*, when the focus is weight loss instead of weight maintenance. When the weight comes off, health improves and other opportunities arise. Although tracking your progress on the scale feels great when you're losing weight, you may also feel the enormous pressure to drop numbers every time you put your feet on the scale.

And when you hit that weight stall, those euphoric feelings can turn into despair if you don't keep yourself grounded. In this chapter we hope to give you a different perspective when it comes down to tracking weight loss and weighing yourself. Here's 3 strategies to stop the scale from asserting so much power of your emotional well-being.

#1 Weight loss as an outcome

Is weight loss the *ultimate* goal? Of course, bariatric surgery is also known as "weight loss surgery". But if we continue to look at weight loss as the main objective, doesn't this automatically trigger distorted behaviors towards the scale?

Because here's the thing.

If weight loss is the main goal, your main focus will be the scale. On top of that, if you've been dieting for years, then it's hard to get out of the "I need to lose weight" mindset. Bariatric surgery may even strengthen that mindset, as weight loss is so apparent in the first months following the surgery. The pressure to lose weight and to focus on how much you weigh can even be amplified further, because of "before and after" pictures on social media and the expectations of your surgeon. The pressure is real.

And that's exactly why we need to raise awareness of this perpetual *(and vicious)* cycle. We want to address that although tracking weight loss is helpful, it should not be the only goal after bariatric surgery. In Chapter 17 we dive deeper into creating new habits and how finding your purpose *(which is more than a number on the scale)*, can be helpful for long-term success.

Keep in mind that we're not discrediting having a goal weight or a target to work towards to. It's helpful for accountability. And there's nothing wrong with taking pride in the weight you've lost. But when you're obsessing over numbers, more than you focus on your daily routines, it's time to take a step back and look at your bariatric journey in the greater light of things. Things such as health improvements, healing your relationship with food and other non-scale victories that bring gratitude.

#2 Why weighing daily is not helpful

Unless you're completely rational, observing and un-emotional when looking at the scale, then weighing yourself daily won't be helpful.

The adrenaline rush when you lose weight is motivating, but the crushing feeling whenever you hit a stall or gain weight – doesn't compare. Your weight fluctuates on a daily basis. And these fluctuations may be entirely unrelated to eating patterns alone. Let's look at 5 things that can cause short-term *(temporary)* weight loss:

- Water retention *(because of sodium intake and glycogen storage)*
- Hormonal factors *(for example, your period is due)*
- Feces weight *(if you didn't have bowel movements for a couple of days – your weight may go up)*
- Differences in muscle mass *(you may be gaining muscles, while losing fat tissue)*
- Sleep deprivation *(leading to less satiety and more cravings the next day)*

But the most important question you might want to ask yourself is this:

"Why do I feel the need to weigh (almost) on a daily basis?"

Tell us if we're wrong here, but it probably has something to do with "feeling in control" right? If you can just see that number going down, then at least you'll have that confirmation that you're on the right track. Weighing daily can become a habit easily if you've tried to lose weight for decades. And only you can decide how often you want to weigh yourself, without feeling anxious about it. You may even decide to stop weighing entirely and only track other progress, like your measurements.

If you're able to separate your emotions from the scale, then we don't see any harm in weighing as often as you want to. But if weighing takes a toll on your mental well-being, it can be truly freeing to stop weighing for a while and shift your focus to your habits entirely, while using another accountability tool to stay the course. The habit tracker in the Bariatric Blueprint freebies *(shared in beginning of this book)* can help you focus on other wins besides weight loss alone.

#3 Focus on what you can control instead of what's out of your hands

You can't control the weather, but you can control what clothes you're going to wear to match today's forecast. And the same applies to your weight loss process too.

When you're following all the basic guidelines, keep up with your new habits and the scale still doesn't move, there isn't anything left to do than staying consistent. Consistency is the hardest when you're doing everything "right", but don't see the results on the scale you were hoping for. Give your body and your habits time to compound. Just because you're not losing weight, doesn't mean that your body isn't preparing to lose weight whenever it's ready again.

Chapter takeaways

- The scale is a helpful tool for accountability and to keep track of your progress overall.
- After bariatric surgery, it's easy to obsess over the number on the scale. Especially if you have been chronically dieting in the past.
- Focusing too much on weight loss outcomes can take away from focusing on new habits.
- When weighing yourself triggers anxiety, it can be helpful to make an agreement with yourself on how often you will weigh – or to refrain from weighing yourself altogether until you get to the root cause of your anxiety.

Chapter 15

Breaking the comparison trap: How to focus on your own success

Changing your mindset after bariatric surgery is a process that requires *introspection*: the ability to look inward for answers instead of looking at what's going on outside of yourself.

One of the distractions from losing sight of what's within, is falling for the notorious comparison trap. The comparison trap can look like comparing your own weight loss progress with others who had surgery around the same date as you. Or perhaps it seems that others don't have as many obstacles as you. Maybe, you feel like other people's journey is *easier* than yours.

Let's start with saying this: there are always going to be other people who lose more weight than you. There are always people with less digestive issues than you may have. But this goes the other way around too. You may have certain advantages that others could only dream of.

Maybe you're incredibly consistent with daily movement. Maybe you are great with meal prepping. And there can be so many other characteristics that are unique to *you*. Things that other people may envy.

Let's get to the point: the comparison trap after bariatric surgery can wreak havoc on the way you feel. And it can open up a can of worms that you really don't want to open *(feelings of envy, jealousy and resentment for example)*.

In this chapter we're giving you 3 key tips to remember every time you feel like you're stumbling into the comparison trap. Let's start breaking the cycle, right here and now.

#1 Stay busy and keep your head down

If you're busy focusing on yourself, you won't have the time to look at what other people are doing. Don't get us wrong. It's more than okay to feel inspired by others within the bariatric community. But what we want to avoid is negative self-talk, feelings of insecurity and other negative emotions when it comes down to looking at other journeys.

A fair question to ask yourself is this:

"What triggers me? What type of stories, results or people make me feel bad about myself?"

Once you get to the bottom of your emotions *(and yes, you have to be really honest about them)*, you discover your own insecurities. And you may discover that these insecurities are often projected into the outside world in the form of "the comparison trap".

The things that you feel secure about, often don't bother you when you see someone else doing them "better". It's the things that you feel insecure about, that trigger the negative spiral of comparison.

It's time to get real. Face your insecurities and own up to them.

In the meantime, stay busy. Focus on your own non-scale victories. Work through letting go of old habits that no longer serve you and replace them with new ones that will help you move forward in your journey. Keep your head down, work hard and become the best version of yourself you can possible be.

#2 Come to terms with what triggers you

Comparing yourself to other people, only to feel bad about yourself afterwards, is often a sign that you desire the thing that these other people seem to have. Maybe you wished you were losing weight quicker, and you see someone else with the same surgery date already hitting their target weight. Perhaps you feel incredibly insecure about your loose skin, and you see somebody who got plastic surgery looking confident through the lens you perceive them with.

The things that trigger you in other people's journey, are often the things that you don't have peace with (yet), within yourself.

It's a harsh truth, but an important one to acknowledge. If you fully come to terms with your insecurities, then you can actively grow stronger from them. Not everything is within your control. Some pieces of your bariatric journey are not fully in your hands, and that can be hard to cope with. Accepting the situation for what it is, can give peace of mind. And finding solutions or inspiration to change the things that you can control, gives more confidence and empowerment.

#3 Gratitude is the key to happiness

Being happy is never an end goal. It's a continuous pursuit of finding gratitude in the small things in life. It's when the things you want, need and wish for, are aligned with what you have. It's having faith that no matter how things look like right now, everything will fall into place eventually; what's meant for you, will come to you.

In other words: it's trusting the process, while finding gratification in the things you do on a daily basis. It's taking a moment to pause, reflect and look around you. Realizing that your life improved in so many ways as opposed to where you once started.

And even if you feel like it hasn't, it's time to take all your setbacks and appreciate them for what they are. Because every hardship you face, makes you stronger. You already proven to yourself that you can do hard things by choosing bariatric surgery. So, how is another setback any different?

Once you feel gratitude in your bariatric journey, *most of the time and despite the hardship* – you're less focused on other people's success in a negative manner. You won't feel upset when someone seems to be making more progress than you.

You are making progress too. Within your own time frame and in your own way.

An important side note is to keep in mind that looks can be very deceiving. Especially on social media platforms where you can only see one side of the story. Remember, that even when somebody shares their "ugly", it can still be highly curated to generate more popularity. Intentions are often hidden when it comes down to social media.

Not all that glitters is gold.

Chapter takeaways

- As a bariatric community, the focus is so often on weight loss and appearance that it's easy to fall for the comparison trap.
- Your own insecurities may be projected onto the outside world, feeling triggered by what other people show – where you feel you're "lacking".
- Ways to keep feelings of envy, jealousy and resentment in check is by staying focused on yourself, coming to terms with your triggers and practice gratitude often and abundantly.

Chapter 16

How to ditch the all-or-nothing mindset

Does making lists like these looks familiar to you?

- "I should eat 80 grams of protein"
- "I should take my vitamins"
- "I should drink my water"
- "I should exercise"
- "I should keep my solids and liquid separate"
- "I should cook more"
- "I should meal prep"
- "I should lose more weight"
- "I should do better"
- "I should *be* better *(wait, am I not good enough?)*"

If the answer is "yes" then this chapter is for you. Here, we're going to share our most valuable insight on ditching the all-or-nothing mindset after bariatric surgery. First, we explain what the "all-or-nothing" mindset looks like. Next, we dive deeper into how you can turn this mindset around. A more flexible mindset to support your life-long journey after bariatric surgery.

The all-or-nothing mindset

The term "all-or-nothing" is pretty straightforward on its own, right? It's either giving your all *(success)*. Or being left with nothing at all *(failure)*. When breaking down the all-or-nothing mindset, it really all boils down to two opposites of a spectrum:

On one end there's everything positive *(accomplished goals, all the wins, all of your success)*. And on the other end, you find an imaginary box where all of failure and misery is buried. The "void" you feel when you didn't meet your goals.

Now, here's the problem.

Life happens. In reality, it's not sustainable to base your outcomes when you hold on to an all-or-nothing mentality. There's nuance everywhere, and that rigid mindset doesn't take that into account.

- Some days you feel good. Some days you don't.
- Some days you have tons of energy. Some days you're drained.
- Some days work is demanding. Some days you can catch a break.

And all of these life events impact your state of mind. They impact your thoughts. They impact how much time you have left in a day. They impact your energy levels.

Simply put: you're not always in control of the things happening to you. Having a rigid mindset isn't going to be helpful here. Not before and also not after bariatric surgery.

What you need is to *grant yourself flexibility*. And a new mindset that supports that flexibility too. When you put *too much pressure* on yourself and have unrealistic expectations, you let the all-or-nothing mindset take over your thoughts and feelings.

But why create goals that won't be sustainable in the long run? Why all the pressure?

The answer is not what you may expect to hear.

It's self-sabotage.

When you set yourself up for failure, you're implying that you don't deserve to be successful. Or, if you never really had any success in your past weight loss experiences, then how are you supposed to know what to do when you *do* succeed? These feelings can be new and overwhelming. And self-sabotage, in a way, protects you from this overwhelm.

But here's the thing.

You *are* destined to do get out of your comfort zone *(otherwise, you wouldn't be brave enough to choose bariatric surgery)*. You can break the cycle of self-sabotage, but you do need to be aware first.

Instead of trying to pursue too many habits that also need to be "perfect" – why not change the action intensity of those habits?

How to stay consistent without being too strict: changing the action intensity

The action intensity of your habits can greatly determine how easy you're making it for yourself to follow through long-term. For example, let's take the topic of "exercise". There are different ways to approach adding exercise to your lifestyle and making it a new habit. You could set this goal for example: *"I'm going to the gym every day at 7 a.m. to do a 60-minute work-out"*.

And you can be great doing that. But then, something comes up. An important deadline from work tying you down. Your child falls ill. Holidays, birthdays and other special occasions that become a distraction. Sometimes, there's just too much going on in your life and you just can't stick to your original plan.

Within an all-or-nothing framework, not showing up like you intend to do *(doing that 60-minute work-out for example)*, feels like an immediate failure. This often results in giving up entirely, because you tie not hitting your goal to a personal failure.

However, a flexible mindset, does allow nuances in your daily routines. This results in still feeling successful, even if you didn't exactly do what you planned on doing.

Here's an example of how you can be more flexible, when it comes down to the initial goal of "doing a 60-minute work-out at 7 a.m.": If you can't make it to the gym at 7 a.m. for whatever valid reason, simplify your main goal. For instance, grab a mat and do 10 sit-ups before starting your day. Instead of beating yourself up for missing your weekly work-out, simply put on your favorite song and dance to it while holding a bottle of water in each hand. It's not always about the extremity of your actions. But more about showing up for yourself, even if it's smaller than you planned initially. But what's even more important, is moving forward in the right direction and doing something (small) that lies in the periphery of your original plan.

(Remember: dancing to one song is way less overwhelming than doing a 60-minute workout at the gym. Sure, you burn more calories doing a 60-minute cardio training, but sometimes settling for something less extreme just to keep the momentum of habit change going, is going to be enough for that busy day.)

Chapter takeaways

- All-or-nothing thinking can stem from feelings of failure, and is a way of self-sabotage on a more unconscious level.
- If there's no space for flexibility, the all-or-nothing mindset takes over.
- Showing up for yourself in small ways is the first step to be more flexible.
- Be okay with not seeing results right away and find peace of mind in the *process* of change itself.

- Giving yourself small rewards when you achieve a new milestone can keep the momentum of change and motivation going.

Chapter 17

New habits: How to rewire your brain after bariatric surgery

Bariatric surgery isn't about losing weight fast. It's about creating *habits* that last.

When the honeymoon stage is over and weight loss comes to a plateau, the habits that you formed in the first couple of months after surgery, are going to be the pillar of the long-term lifestyle change that follows.

This chapter is the core of the mindset work that everyone is talking about after bariatric surgery. The headwork, the mindset "reset" – true personal growth that goes beyond eating your protein and drinking your water.

It's the part of The Bariatric Blueprint where we help you understand how you can change your habits by *rewiring your brain.*

This is probably the hardest part after bariatric surgery as you have to challenge many automated behaviors you may not even be aware of right now.

But don't worry. We're going to break it down for you.

What are habits?

Habits are automated actions that are triggered in response to a cue. For example, brushing your teeth *(automated action)* after waking up *(cue)*. Or washing your hands *(automated action)*, after using the restroom *(cue)*.

Habits exist to make our lives more efficient. We're often not even aware when we act out of habit, because it doesn't require much thinking. Habits help to free up our mental resources for other tasks that do require our full attention.

In psychology, there's a distinction between two types of thinking processes which are used as analogies. There's System 1 which is characterized by fast, automated and intuitive responses. And System 2 is referred to as a more conscious, thoughtful and effortful way of thinking. System 1 thinking occurs fast *(here's where habits play a role)*, while System 2 thinking occurs slow and more deliberate *(here's where changing habits comes to play)*.

Habits are sustained through a so-called "habit loop" and consist out of these 3 basic elements:

The Cue. This is what triggers the habit. Cues could range from anything to location, time, environment or emotional state. The cue is what precedes the automated behavior and what prompts it to occur.
The Routine. This is the actual behavior, or habit, itself.
The Reward. Habits are often sustained because of the perceived value of incorporating that habit. Without a reward, there would be no point in continuing the habit.

Keep in mind that a reward doesn't always have to be beneficial. They could even be harmful, like substance abuse for example.

Let's look at this example in the light of emotional eating as a habit:

The Cue. You didn't get the promotion you worked so hard for. A co-worker ended up getting the promotion and on top of that, took all the credit for your project. You feel sad and angry. The cue here, is emotion: anger and sadness.
The Routine. You're used to "eating away" your emotions. Mostly with sweets. So now, you resort in ice cream for comfort.
The Reward. The instant gratification from eating high-sugar and high-fat ice cream is satisfying, because it affects the pleasure and reward center in the brain *(this part is referred to as the mesolimbic system)*.

Good and bad habits?

Instead of referring to "good" and "bad" habits, we'd like to rephrase this into "helpful" and "unhelpful" habits. By using different language, the morality is removed. And this in turn might help to minimize any self-blame for having "bad" habits.

The helpful habits will assist you in living the life you set out for yourself and being the person, you truly want to be. And the unhelpful habits stray you away from what you truly desire. But even the "bad" habits were helpful at some point. They may have functioned as a coping mechanism when you didn't have the tools to deal with life's challenges in another way. Things that are often called bad habits in light of lifestyle events, like:

- Overeating
- Emotional eating
- Ordering take-out daily
- Eating high-sugar foods after every meal
- Drinking soda
- Going to bed too late

…may have been helpful at some point in life *(again, helpful is not the same as beneficial)*. Perhaps, ordering take-out helped you save time when you were completely overwhelmed. Or drinking soda gave that instant sugar rush, because your brain became dependent on a high-sugar diet. These are part of the so-called rewards as mentioned in the habit loop.

But now it's time to reframe this part. It's time to face the truth. Which habits are going to be replaced for new ones? What automated behaviors do you need to bring to the surface to create new habits instead?

Creating new habits instead of suppressing old ones

"I should stop eating cookies"
"I should stop skipping meals"
"I should stop drinking together with my meals"

These are oversimplified examples of what could potentially happen when you try to change your behavior: restricting yourself into "stop doing something" to get a better outcome.

But here's the thing.

Research shows that suppressing *(inhibiting)* certain unfavored habits, does NOT help in creating new ones. By thinking of not wanting to do something, you're still triggering the old habit, making it harder to replace it with a new one.

But there's hope, because the brain is an amazing organ. Here's where the concept of *neuroplasticity* chimes in.

Neuroplasticity is referred to the brain's ability to form new neural pathways. And this ability is exactly what we need to focus on, when rewiring your brain during your bariatric journey.

Now, let's explain how you can create new habits by reframing your thoughts, beliefs, feelings and ultimately – your actions.

How to rewire your brain: neuroplasticity

Your brain is made out of neurons. And the connections between those neurons are the neural pathways. The longer a habit exists, the more automated the behavior and the stronger the neural pathway becomes.

The key to changing your habits after bariatric surgery, is changing the neural pathways in your brain. Changing your mindset post-op is so much more than simply setting the intention to "do better" starting Monday. It's daily work in the form of affirmations, mindfulness, introspection and awareness. And it takes dedication, commitment and repetition to form those new connections that ultimately are going to be the very root of your new habits.

You can compare your neural pathways with different types of roads. Some roads have been travelled so many times, that there's no denying it leads you from point A to point B – let's call these "the brick roads". And there are other paths that are less travelled, but it's still pretty obvious that you can walk there: like a "hikers' trail".

Other paths are yet to be discovered; nobody knows that there's a way through; this is the starting point of where new habits are formed.

Imagine a forest with bushes, twigs and branches everywhere. It's going to be incredibly hard to break through all the flora. But with continuous effort and the right tools, eventually you'll create a new path. Every time you walk on that lesser-known path, the trail becomes more apparent, until perhaps it even becomes a hikers' trail!

Let's break this down in the context of different habits.

The brick road

The habits that are ingrained in your brain since childhood, exist for decades and are so automated that you're barely aware of them. These are the "brick road habits". These habits require minimal effort and they're triggered easily. It's going to be the hardest to replace these strong wired habits and it will require the most work.

The hikers' trail

These habits are well established and the neural pathways are definitely there. It's hard to break these habits as you've been used to these behaviors for a while now. Luckily, the "hikers' trail" is not so challenging to replace for a new trail, in comparison to the brick road.

The undiscovered path

A new path can be made through different neuroplasticity techniques, which in turn creates new habits. You may not deem it possible to make a new way, but your brain is capable of doing so.

Let's show you how with these 4 techniques.

Creating new habits that stick

Your "Why"

The first step to creating new habits is to have a purpose. The true purpose after bariatric surgery is also referred to as *"your why"*. Keep in mind that your true purpose doesn't have to be reduced to one thing only. There can be numerous reasons why you chose bariatric surgery to improve your life. Write each of those reasons down, and while you do that, make sure to connect with these motivations too. This brings us right to the second technique in creating new habits: visualization.

Visualization

To make a new habit last, you need to hold on to a strong idea in your mind of how life would *look and feel like* with the habits you're going to create. Better said, it's an absolute must to visualize yourself as the person that you want to be.

How would you look like?
How would you feel?
How are you in relation to the loved ones in your life (e.g., what type of mother, friend, daughter, sister, father, brother, etc.), would you be?
What values would you have?
How would you think of yourself?
How would you think of your body?
How would you want other people to describe you?
What would you do on a daily basis?
What would make you happy?
What would make you sad?

These are only a handful of questions to get started for visualizing your best self. Keep in mind that "your best self" isn't an outcome. It's somebody who you can work towards today, and continue to maintain when you get to that point.

Being happy and healthy is a constant pursuit of the new habits you're working on. The bariatric journey doesn't have a "finish line" – it's a continuous recommitment to your beliefs and values.

By visualizing and connecting with your best self, multiple times a day, you're off to a great start forming those new neural pathways.

The power of feeling

Research shows that neural pathways are strengthened when emotions are connected to our thoughts. Visualization may be the fuel, but connecting your emotions will ignite the process of changing your habits. To replace a new habit with an old one, you have to imagine how you would feel when performing the new habit. Let's say you want to replace the habit of "watching tv after dinner" with "walking after dinner". The first step in the process would be to define your purpose. Why do you want to walk after dinner instead of binge-watching your favorite series?

Your purpose may be that you want to feel energetic. Or perhaps you want to reap the benefits of increasing your physical strength.

Next, you want to visualize how this will go. You can choose whether you reserve a specific time in the day for visualization exercises, like after waking up, or before going to bed (or both!). During this visualization exercise, you picture yourself having dinner, cleaning the dishes and putting on your walking shoes. You imagine the path you're going to walk, or even just walking a block around the house. The key is to truly see yourself walking outside and doing what you intend to do. Next, it's time to connect a feeling to this picture. Perhaps, you can almost smell the fresh air making you feel energized. Or you feel a light breeze against your cheeks, relieving you from the stress at work. Maybe you feel a sense of pride for accomplishing what you set out to do.

The power of feeling is not only appreciating your feelings afterwards, but also *before* you actually perform the behavior.

Repetition is key

Okay, now that we have 3 techniques covered, finding your purpose, visualization and connecting your feelings, we need to move on to the most difficult challenge of them all: repetition.

The more often you repeat your favored behavior *(your new habit)*, the stronger the neural pathway becomes. Here's where your undiscovered trail becomes a hikers' trail and perhaps even a brick road in due time.

Through repetitive actions, you become more familiar with the new behavior. Again, suppressing your old patterns and behaviors isn't going to be helpful. Here's where having a plan comes in handy.

When are you going to perform the desired behavior?
Are there other people involved in performing your new habits (perhaps a walking-buddy)?
How long are you going to partake in the new behavior?

The more detailed your plan, the higher the likelihood of following through. Here, it's also incredibly important to set realistic expectations, because setting the bar too high happens so easy, right? Remember the all-or-nothing mentality we talked about in the previous chapters? Well, this is exactly how an all-or-nothing mindset can sabotage your new habits: by setting the bar so high that it becomes nearly impossible to sustain your new patterns of behavior. Simply put: having an all-or-nothing mindset is self-sabotage in the process of change.

Things to keep in mind

Change is always easier said than done. Even though we've laid down the basics of creating new habits, the task itself isn't a walk in the park. How to get out of your own way is the greatest riddle to solve when you're trying to improve yourself. Here's what you can expect when doing the real mindset work:

Uncomfortable and awkward

When you unravel your own behavior and challenge yourself to face the reasons why you do what you do and don't do what you want to do – you may feel greatly uncomfortable. Dealing with feelings can be incredibly hard. Also, let's not forget about the feelings of failure, self-judgment or even self-loathing when you think of every attempt to better your life, but still feel like you're back at square one.

We need to reframe this way of thinking.

The only way to truly change is to become more compassionate toward yourself. And to forgive yourself for not knowing better in the past. You have to move beyond the feelings of shame and failure, to move forward. Nobody is perfect, and you don't have to be either. Looking at your behavior as an observer instead of a judge, is crucial to take the steps mentioned in this chapter.

Familiarity and the path of least resistance

When changing habits, we have to take the "familiarity effect" into account. This effect is referred to as an automatic preference for the things that are familiar to us. Again, familiarity isn't necessarily beneficial. But even if the familiar is harmful, we may still hold a preference towards it. For example, imagine coming from a household where both parents are narcissists. Toxic traits, such as neglect, gaslighting and manipulation, were the "normal" in this home. If you're not aware of these mechanisms and don't have the tools to heal, then chances are that you'll be attracting the exact same traits that were harmful being a child, later on when seeking a partner in life.

What's familiar, becomes normal. What's normal, feels more comfortable. And that's why it's absolutely necessary to step out of your comfort zone when changing your entire lifestyle. Step by step, at your own pace. Pull away out of your comfort zone too brass, and it may backfire. But not taking action at all, is definitely not going to be helpful.

Besides preferring familiarity, we also prefer the *path of least resistance* when it comes down to taking action. We automatically gravitate to things that don't require much effort. This is biology's way of preserving our energy levels for times when we do need to take action quickly. And this again, boils down to getting comfortable with being uncomfortable. And to fully accept that the results you're seeking for, can lag. You may lose all hope and motivation when you don't see results after all the work you've been putting in. But we have to acknowledge that even if you can't see anything changing, underneath the surface, the process of change is in full effect. Allow your daily habits to result into a compound effect, fuelled by repetition and consistency.

Reframing thoughts: Journaling and affirmations

Are you staring back at your reflection feeling proud and accomplished? Or are you avoiding every mirror because you "hate" the way you look?

Your thoughts predict your feelings. And your feelings impact your actions. In order to reframe your thought processes, you may have to dig deeper and challenge some of the beliefs you've been holding (about yourself) for way too long.

Some beliefs, are false beliefs:

"I'm a failure"
"I can never get anything right"
"I'm always miserable"
"My surgery failed"
"I can't stick to anything"

…are just a handful examples of false beliefs that further amplify automated negative thoughts, making it so much more challenging to change your mindset. If you continue to look at yourself from a point of self-judgment, success is going to be far out of reach.

It's time to challenge yourself, face your insecurities and reframe automated negative thoughts into accurate thoughts.

How do you start this process? How can you change the way you think?

Well, first we need to bring the thoughts to light. If they remain hidden in your subconscious, you may never even know they're there.

Second, journaling can provide clarity and an overview of all the thoughts and feelings inside. They make your thoughts more tangible as opposed to being tiny snippets of information that appear briefly, only to disappear in your subconscious again.

Third, positive affirmations can change the way you think. Positive affirmations help you "unbelieve" false thoughts and create more accurate ones. Let's look at a few examples:

Table 5. Reframing thought processes after bariatric surgery

Negative thought	Reframing + problem-solving thinking
I'm a failure	I'm not perfect, but I'm not giving up. I'm still learning. And that's okay.
I never meet my protein goals	I didn't meet my protein goal today. How can I increase my protein intake? What do I need to change in my diet? Do I need to eat more frequently? Do I need to make different food choices? Do I need to talk to my dietitian?
I don't have time to meal prep	I didn't prioritize meal prepping today, because I had other important things to do. I will prioritize meal prepping tomorrow. What can I do to get started?
I can't do anything right	Sometimes I make mistakes, this is part of being human. How can I stop sabotaging myself? Why am I getting in my own way?
I'll never reach my goal weight	I didn't reach my goal weight *yet*. On what other goals, besides weight loss, can I focus right now?

	What can I do right now, do act upon the new habits I created?
I can't stick to my plan	I didn't follow my plan today. What were the obstacles? How can I overcome these hurdles? Do I need to set the bar a little lower to make this plan more realistic and sustainable?

It's important to keep in mind that "the mindset work" may require additional tools like (cognitive-behavioral) therapy or other interventions like meditation. What works for you, may not work for somebody else. Always consult your healthcare provider if you need further guidance in this area.

Chapter takeaways

- Habits are automated actions that are ingrained in our brain.
- Suppressing old habits doesn't seem to be helpful in creating new ones.
- Creating new habits is possible through the concept of neuroplasticity.
- Finding purpose, visualization, connecting feelings, repetition, reframing thoughts and journaling are techniques to help create new habits that stick.

Part 5

Get unstuck after weight stalls and weight regain

Chapter 18

Why your weight is stalling and what (not) to do about it

Weight stalls during your weight loss phase after bariatric surgery can be terribly disheartening. You're losing weight for weeks and then all of the sudden, your weight loss comes to a halt and you hit that infamous plateau *(or multiple ones, back-to-back)*.

In this chapter, we get into the nitty-gritty of weight stalls and whether there's something you can actively do, and if it's necessary in the first place, to break your weight stall. So, keep on reading if you want to know what to do next time the scale isn't moving.

Why weight stalls are so frustrating after bariatric surgery

But first let's start with why weight stalls feel like a "slap in the face" after bariatric surgery. To answer this question, we have to go back to the pre-op days when you tried every diet in the books to lose weight. The diets didn't work. Not long-term at least. And now, bariatric surgery is your "last chance" for weight loss and improved health. This means that a lot of pressure is built over the years and "losing weight" may even became part of your identity. You can't remember a day in your life when you were NOT trying to lose weight.

This creates pressure. Lots of pressure.

The pressure to lose weight. The pressure to not regain. The pressure to create new habits. And the list goes on and on. Add toxic diet culture on top of that and you have the perfect recipe for a mindset where you're probably being way too harsh on yourself. And this mindset only leads to feelings of failure and continuous disappointment. Bariatric surgery is a medical intervention to treat the physical implications of obesity, but it's not a surgery on your thoughts and feelings.

And the way your feelings are triggered by a weight stall, well, they're related to your mindset too! So, before we dive into the physiological, nutritional and hormonal part of weight stalls, we want to make this one thing perfectly clear:

Weight stalls are normal. They're a part of your weight loss journey. They will happen and you're not a failure if you're not losing weight at the same rate all the time.

You will enter a phase in your journey where you hit your "weight set point", a specific weight-range where your body feels most comfortable with. You may enter multiple weight set points the closer you get to your goal weight, or when you're entering the maintenance stage of your bariatric journey.

With that being said let's start with one of the most important nutritional factors why you may stop losing weight: insufficient protein intake.

The link between weight stalls, weight loss and protein after bariatric surgery

Protein is the building block of your muscles. And we explained in Chapter 8 why bariatric surgery puts you at risk for the loss of muscle mass.

Your muscle mass growth is dependent on things such as:

- Protein intake
- Physical activity
- Age and gender

If you lose muscle mass, your metabolism slows down. And this could potentially lead to slower weight loss. Always remember to eat your protein first and to keep a close eye on your protein goals as you progress through your journey.

Getting your fluids in is invaluable for healthy weight loss after bariatric surgery. Sipping all day long and still nowhere near your hydration goals? We get it, it's not an easy task to stay hydrated when you can't eat and drink at the same time or when water makes you nauseous.

But we can't forget about the basics.

You need liquids to keep all basic bodily functions working properly. But hydration also plays a key role in a solid working metabolism. When your metabolism is up and running, it will be easier to lose weight as well.

Lack of sleep can lead you straight into a weight stall

Sleep deprivation is often underestimated when it comes down to weight stalls *(and even weight gain)*. Poor sleep quality or lack of sleep is linked to an increase in your hunger hormones *(ghrelin)* and a decrease in the hormones that make you feel full longer *(leptin)*. When you're sleep deprived, your ghrelin levels rise and your leptin levels drop. Simply put: you're crave more energy through food which could lead to overeating.

Hunger hormones play an important role in regulating appetite and ultimately in the food choices you make. Also, when you're tired you may find yourself craving more slider foods like sweets, chips and chocolate. Creating an intentional evening routine may help you improve your sleep pattern.

Mindless grazing can be another tricky pitfall

Have you ever wondered why it's so easy to eat a bowl of chips, but you're struggling to eat a few pieces of chicken? To answer this question, it's important that you're aware of the nutrient density of different food sources.

Now, chips and chicken are not the same. One is a slider food while the other is a high-protein food source. Slider foods such as popcorn, chips, pretzels, cookies and ice cream are typically easier to digest because they're high in carbohydrates and low in protein and/or fiber. Digestion of slider foods already starts in your mouth with an enzyme called *amylase* found in your saliva. Protein doesn't start to digest until it's in your pouch with the help of an enzyme called *protease*. Slider foods leave your pouch faster than nutrient dense foods, therefore not keeping your small stomach full for long. It's easy to overeat on slider foods, especially when you're already struggling to eat a high-protein, high-fiber meal. The reason why you're struggling to eat non-slider food meals, may because of:

- High restriction *(you're simply too full)*
- Digestive issues *(like nausea)*

That's why it's so much easier to graze on slider foods after bariatric surgery. And bringing this to light, is key to understanding certain eating patterns. Now, if mindless grazing becomes a pitfall, keep these strategies in mind:

- Whenever you eat something, put your food on a plate *(or in a bowl)* first. Avoid eating straight from the package.
- Plan your meals and snacks. Having a plan isn't a guarantee that you'll stick to it every single time, but it does help.
- Add high-protein and/or a high-fiber food sources to your snacks to keep you full for longer. Foods that are also high in unsaturated fats, such as avocados, keep you satisfied too.
- Have a kind conversation with yourself. Whenever you have the urge to nibble on slider foods, tell

yourself that it's okay to have these cravings. And ask yourself this question: Why am I craving this right now? Am I hungry? Am I tired? Am I stressed? Am I sad? Am I doing this out of habit? Once you start to unravel the reasons behind the craving, you can observe the urge without the self-loathing part and preferably with lots of self-compassion.

Don't think weight loss – but think in healthy body composition instead

Not all weight loss is the same. If you lose muscle mass, you may be losing weight on the scale, but at the end of the day, your metabolism takes a hit.

Losing fat tissue is what we're aiming for, especially after bariatric surgery where the preservation of your muscle mass is already at risk. When you maintain an active lifestyle over time, you're promoting muscle maintenance. And depending on what type of exercise you're doing, maybe even muscle growth. Next time you hit a plateau, make sure to track your measurements too.

If you're losing inches, this can indicate that you're losing fat mass. You may see a "stall" in total body weight, but when you simultaneously gaining muscle mass, it's actually beneficial for your overall body composition.

The 3-week stall explained

Everyone loses weight at a different rate after bariatric surgery, but there seems to be one common denominator: the 3-week stall. What happens around 3 weeks post-op? And why is it so common for weight loss to plateau all of the sudden? Well, the answer has everything to do with your glycogen storage.

Glucose is stored as glycogen in your muscles and liver. But when you've been on liquids for the first few weeks after bariatric surgery *(and followed the low-carb, liver shrinking diet before bariatric surgery too)*, your body's glycogen storage is most likely (almost) all used up.

But after a few weeks in, you slowly start to add more foods and textures to your diet, meaning that you're refueling the glycogen storage in your liver and muscles. Glycogen binds to water causing "weight gain". This in turn leads to a temporary stall in weight loss.

On top of that, your body is also adjusting to major changes which may cause hormones to fluctuate, hindering weight loss (temporary).

Weight stall or weight maintenance: weight set point

How do you know whether you hit (another) stall, or that you're entering the maintenance phase of your bariatric journey? To answer that question, we need to explain more about the *weight set point.*

Your weight set point refers to the weight your body "feels most comfortable with" and is regulated by all sorts of metabolic processes. It's a weight range of about 5-20 pounds that is predetermined, so that our body can exist in complete balance *(homeostasis)*. Through the change of gut hormones (and mechanisms that aren't fully understood yet), bariatric surgery changes your weight set point – making it "easier" to maintain a certain weight at a lower range than before surgery.

But your weight set point may also work against your goals. Biology has its own way of creating balance, and this may not always be aligned with the specific weight target you set out. If your goal weight is lower than your weight set point, it's going to be harder to lose the last pounds: your body is literally doing everything in its power not to lose weight any more.

Being aware of the fact that you have a weight set point to begin with, creates more self-compassion and understanding of why your weight may be stalling *(for so long)*.

The strategy to lowering your weight set point so that you continue your weight loss process, is staying consistent in the new habits you create today. There's no magic, just helpful habits repeated over a longer period of time.

Medical reasons for slower weight loss and weight stalls

Weight stalls aren't just related to what you eat and how you eat. We already discussed the impact of your weight set point. But there's also something else to take into account when looking at slower weight loss: medical conditions that hinder the weight loss process.

When bariatric surgery leads to weight loss, co-morbidities may improve or even resolve. Some bariatric patients with diabetes report not needing their insulin any longer as shortly as a few days after their surgery. Losing weight can also lead to improvements in blood pressure, blood lipids, cholesterol levels and joint issues. Just to name a few of many more benefits.

However, bariatric surgery is not a cure-all for all co-morbidities and underlying medical conditions. For example, the symptoms of chronic diseases like PCOS (polycystic ovarian syndrome) and hypothyroidism, may still linger after bariatric surgery. The impact of these endocrine disorders may not fully dissolve with losing weight after bariatric surgery and therefore, can impact your weight loss outcomes too.

Chapter takeaways

Weight stalls after bariatric surgery are normal. You're not failing your surgery if you hit a plateau. A few things to double-check when you hit a stall are these:

- Adding protein.
- Drinking water *(or low-calorie/zero-calorie liquids if you can't tolerate water).*
- Being physically active.
- Keeping mindless grazing in check.

- Remaining consistent while following the basic principles. The input of your work doesn't always match the output on the scale right away. Results often lag.
- Stop relying on your motivation to build habits, but rather, focus on finding joy and discipline in daily routines. It's cliché, because it works.
- Asking for guidance from your bariatric team or a certified health practitioner to discuss your personal needs.

Chapter 19

Weight regain: beyond the shame

Before we dive into the topic of weight regain, let's start with saying that weight regain deserves so much more depth, than the feelings of failure it's often associated with. Weight regain is not uncommon after bariatric surgery. And it's only when we disconnect the shame from gaining weight after losing it, we can find solutions to make things better. So, let's start with the feelings, before we move forward with the answers.

The emotions behind weight regain: feelings of failure

Shame.

The shame of failing your surgery.
The shame of failing yourself.

It's okay to be frank about your emotions after weight regain. But it's even more important to question whether the shame regarding your regain is accurate.

Let's explain.

A bit of weight regain after bariatric surgery is expected. Remember, the 5–20-pound range when we explained the weight set point in the previous chapter? A bit of weight regain may be expected if we take this range into account.

Now, what do the statistics say? Well, the number of bariatric patients that experience weight regain differ from study to study. And the reason why is that there doesn't seem to be a unanimous definition when it comes down to describing exactly what regain is. Taking this into account, the range of bariatric patients that experience weight regain is between 16-37%.

In our book *The Big Reset,* we go into the depths on how to tackle weight regain. But because this topic is so important, we felt obliged to dedicate a chapter on weight regain in this book. Let's start with possible causes for weight regain.

Causes for weight regain

There can be different causes for the scale to trickle up again after you've lost the weight initially. And a few of those reasons are related to the basic principles of a bariatric lifestyle. They're not new. You've heard about them. You've practiced them. And we talked about the bariatric basics throughout this entire book. But to refresh your memory, here are a handful of basic principles to fall back on, whenever you feel stuck:

- Prioritize your protein
- Stay hydrated

- Take your vitamins
- Keep solids from liquids
- Avoid refined sugars
- Work on your relationship with food
- Keep yourself accountable
- Go to your follow-up appointments
- Do your blood work
- Move your body in a way that's sustainable
- Chew well and eat slow
- Understand your non-hunger cues
- Find gratitude in your journey, despite the challenges
- Celebrate your scale and non-scale victories

When you lose sight of these basic principles, you may find yourself straying away from your purpose – *your why*. When you go through the motions of weight regain, it can be helpful to ask yourself the following questions:

1. What habits that I practiced before, are fading away now?
2. How did my mental well-being change over the past couple of months?
3. Did something drastic happened recently? *(For example: new job, having a baby or the loss of a loved one).*
4. Do I need help from a therapist, dietitian, personal trainer or another (healthcare) professional to set up a new plan to work on my health? What specifically am I struggling with right now?

5. Do I still hold myself accountable? Am I aware of my own behavior, or am I on auto-pilot?

It's never too late to start again. Even though bariatric surgery is called a "last resort", it's not your "last chance". Changing habits and dealing with the chronic illness of obesity, is hard. And it's okay to need more time to re-evaluate your goals and the direction you're heading to.

Grazing and weight regain

Grazing is referred to as eating small amounts of (slider) foods over a longer period of time. When you graze, you're less inclined to eat wholesome balanced meals throughout the day. Not-so-fun-fact: grazing can easily lead to overeating.

On top of that, grazing is associated with "loss of control eating" or LOCE. An eating pattern that's related to several eating disorders, like binge eating disorder. When you experience LOCE you lose track of time and you don't notice your fullness cues as well as opposed to when you eat more mindful.

Grazing is one of the top eating habits that lead to weight regain after bariatric surgery. Creating awareness is necessary to tackle this issue.

Unresolved emotional issues and mental health issues

When you feel good, it's easier to do better. And if you don't feel good, discipline must be greater than motivation alone. But that is easier said than done.

When you suffer from mental health issues, food can be an outlet in many ways. Maybe food has become and remains a coping mechanism after bariatric surgery. Or perhaps your mental health makes it harder to stick to "basic rules" such as meal planning. The topic of mental health is vast. The key point here is to remind you to take care of yourself in more ways than simply "eating your protein and drinking your water".

Dig deeper. Go the extra mile. Explore what's keeping you from being the best version you can possibly be.

Go the extra mile: explore why you're sabotaging yourself

Self-sabotaging behaviors aren't always obvious. For example, procrastination protects against failure: if you delay your actions, you never fail. The downside of course, is that you never succeed either.

To get started with bringing self-sabotage to light, you can ask yourself the following questions:

1. If there would be zero limitations and anything would be possible, what do you want in your life that you don't have right now *(not just weight loss related)*?
2. What scares you the most when visualizing yourself being *there*?
3. What are you telling yourself when you want something, but don't have it yet?

It's the things you're most afraid of, that need to be faced. Step by step. Layer by layer. Change never happens when you're comfortable. It's when you challenge yourself, *emotionally*, you learn exactly why you keep getting in your own way.

It won't be pretty. Healing is hard and confronting. But this part of the process is necessary for growth. The fear of failure is real. Especially after bariatric surgery when you already put so much pressure on yourself to *really make it work this time around*. The fear of failure is further increased by the self-distrust that has been built up through "failed" attempts to lose weight and most of all – keep it off. Because every time you tried to lose weight and it didn't work out, it spirals you in a state of distrust. And the despair can be debilitating. It's going to take time and intentional effort to rebuild that self-trust again. Giving up is not an option!

Chapter takeaways

- Weight regain happens in up to 37% of bariatric patients and is often associated with feelings of failure and shame.
- Things that can help to manage regain are the following:
- Eat wholesome and nutritious meals to prevent grazing; focus on protein, fiber and unsaturated fats.
- Prevent grazing by putting your food on a plate. Avoid eating straight from a package. It's harder to create portion control when you can't see how much you're eating.

- Work on your root causes for emotional eating; what exactly are you trying to suppress with food? Why are you distracting yourself with food? What makes you want to get that "rush" from eating? Remember, you don't have to find all these answers on your own. A therapist can help you with this part of your journey too.
- Be sure to maintain an active lifestyle that works for you over time. "Trends" may sound fun, but sustainability over popularity – any time.
- Don't skip your follow-up appointments. If you can't make it, always reschedule. There's a direct correlation between poor follow-up care/commitment and weight regain.
- Avoid high-calorie liquids as they easily slide through your stomach and don't do anything for your restriction.
- Focus on changing your daily habits, instead of restricting yourself into a "dieting" mentality. One habit at a time, one day at a time. Small steps go a long way. And remember: you don't have to hit your goal weight at 12 months post-op. The journey to healing and self-growth doesn't have a deadline. Drop the pressure and continue to show up for yourself in small ways.
- Be honest about the ways you're sabotaging your own progress. Are you scared of success? Are you afraid you will fail once you get what you really want? Do you believe you are deserving of all the things you wish for? Dig deep and do the soul-searching. Embrace the "suck".

Chapter 20

Pouch stretching: myths and facts

Pouch stretching and stoma dilation. What are the myths and what exactly, are the facts? Do you really need to worry about stretching your stomach every time you can eat more than before? The good news is that pouch stretching after bariatric surgery is less common than the fear itself.

But first, let's address this question:

"Why is stomach stretching a common fear after bariatric surgery?"

Let's get into it: The fear of pouch stretching

There's one common denominator in all bariatric journeys: bariatric surgery is one of many tools to fight the debilitating chronic disease called "obesity". When you feel restricted in what you eat, your portions decrease and you see the scale go down every time you step on it – it's nothing but sheer euphoria.

Losing weight and maintaining a healthy weight didn't work before *(yes, we're talking about trying to lose weight with all those countless diets that didn't help you long-term)*. And now, your hard work finally pays off.

So, it makes perfect sense that the moment your portions increase, doubt kicks in. Maybe you didn't expect to eat more *this* soon. Or maybe you expected your appetite to come back, but just not *this* strongly.

Whatever the reason, you feel like you can't risk "failing your surgery": the pressure is at an all-time high.

And here's where we need to stop you in your tracks for a moment.

Once you acknowledge these fears and the feeling of insecurities that go hand-in-hand with increased portions, an ever-fluctuating appetite and the scale that doesn't seem to do what you want – it's time for a mindset change.

Here's where confidence *(trusting the process)*, consistency and self-trust come into play.

Understanding how nutrition affects your portions and appetite, is key in easing the fear around pouch stretching. Besides nutrition, you also need to be aware of the basic anatomy of your stomach.

The anatomy of your pouch after bariatric surgery

Bariatric surgery resizes your stomach to about 20% of its original size. Immediately after surgery, your pouch is still swollen. This means that part of your restriction is caused by the swelling in your stomach. Once the swelling subsides, you're more likely to increase your portions.

Your stomach is designed to naturally stretch when holding a meal, and shrink back whenever the food passes to the rest of your digestive system. You can compare this to the stretching and shrinking of an accordion.

The reason why, is because your stomach's lining is made out of muscular tissue, called the *rugae*. These muscles are needed to make sure that you can hold a meal as they expand when your stomach fills up.

But how do you know whether you stretched your stomach or not?

The only way to accurately determine whether your pouch has stretched to the extent that it impacts your bariatric weight loss journey in a negative manner, is through an endoscopy or barium swallow test performed by a licensed medical specialist. Tests like these can determine whether you have stretched your pouch or dilated your stoma *(the passage between your pouch and your small intestine)*. "Do It Yourself" pouch stretching tests are not reliable.

Rest assured; stomach stretching is far less likely than that it's feared. Oftentimes, you may think you have stretched your stomach because you can eat more. But this isn't a reliable measurement. You're supposed to eat more food (volume) once you're further out of surgery. This is a completely normal part of the process after bariatric surgery.

But we do need to be mindful of one pitfall: overeating.

The link between overeating and stretching your pouch

Even though your stomach is supposed to stretch when you're eating *(otherwise the food would have no space at all)*, this doesn't mean that you can't stretch your stomach beyond the norm. It's totally valid to wonder *what causes* stomach stretching in the first place?

Well, the main reason probably doesn't surprise you. It's consistently overeating beyond your fullness cues. And here are a few examples that make overeating more likely:

- When you eat past your fullness cues
- When you ignore your fullness cues altogether
- When you graze on slider foods continuously without a long-term solution at hand
- When you don't separate your solids from your liquids any longer
- When you eat too fast
- When you fall prey to problematic emotional eating (e.g., binge eating)
- When you experience chronic stress and resort to food as a coping mechanism

- When you're chronically sleep deprived and use food as a means to stay energized
- When you're not meeting your protein and fiber goals long-term

If you're oblivious to the mechanisms that potentially trigger overeating, then it becomes so much harder to brace yourself for these patterns. And if you remember well, we discussed the strategies to prevent overeating in chapter 10. Make sure to return back to these strategies as often as you need.

The illusion of pouch stretching

Portion size is only valuable if we look at the context of the meal. Not all meals are created equal. A full breakfast plate of Oreo cookies isn't the same as a full breakfast plate of chicken breast and broccoli. They may be the same in volume (size), but the nutrient density and the way the meals are being digested, are completely different.

Slider foods, like the cookies, can be eaten in larger quantities because it takes longer to reach your fullness cues. Foods with refined sugars that have little protein, fiber or unsaturated fats – can be eaten in larger volumes. On the other hand, protein dense foods like chicken breast and high-fiber foods like broccoli – are nutrient dense. That meal will take longer to digest and you reach your fullness cues quicker.

The sensation of being able to eat larger amounts of slider foods, gives the false impression that you have stretched your stomach. You haven't stretched your stomach; the food simply is digested quicker, leaving room for more.

But when you eat nutrient dense meals, your restriction is higher. This gives the sensation that your stomach is "small".

So, next time you're afraid of pouch stretching, analyze what meals or foods you ate that made you fearful. And remember that increasing your portions after bariatric surgery is normal and necessary for proper nourishment.

Chapter takeaways

- Pouch stretching and stoma dilation is possible through consistent overeating.
- However, the fear of pouch stretching is often taken out of proportion compared to the likelihood of actually stretching your stomach.
- Some foods may make it seem like you stretched your stomach because they are digested quicker.
- Nutrient dense meals result in higher restriction and a quicker sensation of fullness.

Chapter 21

The truth about "pouch resets" after bariatric surgery

We started this book with explaining that restrictive dieting doesn't work long-term. And now that we came to the final section of The Bariatric Blueprint, we need to bring awareness to that one thing that can lead you straight back into the negative spiral of all-or-nothing thinking and a dieting mentality.

We're talking about "pouch reset diets".

Let's explain why pouch reset diets aren't helpful after bariatric surgery, and what you can do instead to keep the momentum of (weight loss) change going.

What is a pouch reset diet?

Pouch reset diets are liquid diets that mimic the first stages of your post-operative diet. They often consist of protein shakes and other low-calorie liquids only. They're popular within certain subgroups within the bariatric community as a way to break a weight stall, accelerate weight loss or tackle weight regain.

Do they work?

Just like any other fad diet, they bring you in a calorie deficit. And if you burn more calories than you consume, the result is weight loss. But just like any other diet, they don't work long-term.

On top of that, they falsely claim to shrink back your stomach – which is anatomically not possible. There's no reset button to make your stomach as small as right after your surgery. The harsh truth is once again: diets don't work to sustain long-term weight loss. If it didn't work before bariatric surgery, then restrictive dieting won't work after weight loss surgery neither.

The tricky part about pouch reset diets it that they bring you back into a "dieting mentality". And a pouch reset may give you the false impression that you're "back in control" again.

But there's a catch. And it's a big one too.

Pouch resets can cause malnourishment when done without any medical supervision. Your calorie intake may be too low and there's the risk of not getting enough nutrients from liquids only. In that sense, pouch resets aren't only unhelpful but they can be dangerous too.

On top of that, pouch reset diets don't address any underlying causes for weight loss issues. They don't give you the tools to work on consistency and your mindset. Not surprisingly, there's no scientific evidence that pouch reset diets work long-term. But, there's one exception when going back to liquids makes sense.

Medical reasons for a liquid diet

There is one exception in which a liquid diet is helpful after bariatric surgery *(apart from the mandatory post-operative diet of course)*. Pouch resets may be advised in the medical field in case of obstruction or *stenosis*. In other words, going back to liquids may be medically necessary if there's a "road block" in your digestive system making it challenging to allow food to pass through.

Liquid diets should only be advised in the light of a medical reason and supervised by a healthcare professional.

Chapter takeaways

- Pouch reset diets to "shrink back your stomach" are a false claim.
- Pouch reset diets don't fix any underlying reasons why you may be falling off track.
- If you truly want to focus on your goals consistently – and change your mindset along with it – then here's what you to consider instead:
- Reach out to your bariatric team for personal guidance.
- Go back to the bariatric basics: protein, hydration, vitamins, exercise, sleep, self-care and focus on one small goal at a time.
- Start using a bariatric journal to actually keep track of your basics so you can keep yourself accountable.
- Log your food without counting your calories meticulously. Track what you eat to gain insight in

your eating pattern. This way, you may discover on what areas to focus more on.

- Focus more on healing your relationship with food and continue the mindset work.

Moving forward after bariatric surgery

It's time to wrap it up. The Bariatric Blueprint gave you a basic roadmap of what to expect after bariatric surgery and how nutrition and mindset strategies must work together to make your bariatric journey work for you. Bariatric surgery is so much more than following a set of guidelines. Sure, prioritizing your protein and drinking your water are non-negotiables. But the mindset hurdles, dealing with setbacks and getting out of your own way – are key elements to change your mindset so that following the guidelines becomes easier.

Long-term success is what you deserve, and bariatric surgery is an important tool in your toolbox to make that happen.

Celebrating your 1-year Surgiversary is memorable. However, your bariatric journey doesn't have a deadline. You don't have to hit all of your goals in your honeymoon stage. And you decide how you show up for yourself to make your bariatric journey work. Because, building a new lifestyle when you're eating habits change, is hard. But that won't stop you from doing what needs to be done.

The *continuous commitment* you promised yourself the day you set foot in that surgery room, is the key to your success. And we truly hope that this book unlocked more knowledge, instilled hope and gave you the motivation to continue to move forward.

Don't stop. Don't give up. And remember, that there's always a community *(yes, Your Onederland)* you can rely on. We're wishing you all the best in this life-changing journey to become who you truly want to be. May you be able to celebrate all your non-scale victories and embrace the soul-searching that comes along with changing your life. You got this!

More bariatric resources and a free community platform

- Learn more about our community on www.youronederland.com.
- Get more than 40 bariatric friendly recipes on www.bari-tasty.com.
- Loved this book? There's more! Check out our signature bariatric book collection on www.youronederland.com/all-bariatric-books

Spread the word!

We love creating new bariatric resources for the community, but we need your help to spread the word. If you enjoyed The Bariatric Blueprint, please leave a review on Amazon. We'd appreciate it so much!

Bariatric glossary

We listed the most common abbreviations, terminology and definitions used in the field of bariatric surgery and within the bariatric community below.

Abbreviations for bariatric surgery procedures

(L)AGB	(laparoscopic) adjustable gastric banding, referring to a device being placed around the top of the stomach which creates a small pouch above the band.
BPD/DS	biliopancreatic diversion with duodenal switch, refers to a mixed bariatric surgery procedure where a part of the stomach is removed and about 75% of the small intestine is bypassed.
EGS	endoscopic sleeve gastroplasty, refers to a minimal invasive bariatric procedure where a suturing device is inserted into the throat reducing the size of the stomach. No incisions are made.
MGB	mini gastric bypass, refers to the gastric bypass procedure which involves only one connection as opposed to the traditional gastric bypass which involves multiple rerouting.

RYGB/RGB/GB	roux-en-y gastric bypass, refers to a mixed bariatric procedure where a part of the stomach and the small intestine are bypassed.
SADI-S	single anastomosis duodeno-ileal bypass with sleeve gastrectomy, refers to the bariatric procedure where about 80% of the stomach is removed (similar to the gastric sleeve) and the latter part of the small intestine is connected to the stomach. There's only one connection.
VSG/SG	vertical sleeve gastrectomy, refers to the bariatric procedure where about 80% of the stomach is removed.
WLS	weight loss surgery, refers to all weight loss surgery procedures to treat obesity.

Other abbreviations

BMR	basic metabolic rate, the number of calories needed to maintain basic bodily functions.
CW	current weight.
CPAP	continuous positive airway pressure, refers to a breathing therapy device to treat sleep

	apnea – a common comorbidity before bariatric surgery.
EWL	excess weight loss, can be determined by subtracting your current weight from your ideal weight.
GERD	gastroesophageal reflux disease, occurs when stomach acid repeatedly flows back into the esophagus
GLP-1	glucagon-like peptide 1, refers to a hormone produced by the intestinal L-cells in response to glucose and other ingested nutrients. It delays the emptying of the stomach and enhances insulin secretion.
GW	goal weight, refers to target weight.
HW	highest weight, refers to the highest weight ever recorded
LCD	low-calorie diet, refers to the diet prior to bariatric surgery in order to shrink the liver. The LCD is typically around 800 calories a day.
LRD/LSD	liver reduction diet/liver shrinking diet, refers to the low-fat and low-calorie diet prior to surgery in order to shrink the liver size to prevent complications such as bleeding during surgery.

LW	lowest weight, refers to the lowest weight ever recorded
NSV	non-scale victory, refers to all successes besides losing weight as seen on the scale.
PAL	physical activity level, refers to a way to express daily activity level as a number. And is used to estimate total energy expenditure.
PPI	proton pump inhibitors, refers to medication to reduce the amount of stomach acid being produced by the glands in the stomachs' lining.
PYY	peptide YY, refers to the hunger hormone that helps to reduce appetite and limit food intake. PYY is produced mainly in the last part of the gastro-intestinal tract.
SW	surgery weight, refers to the weight on surgery day
SX	surgery.
TEE	total energy expenditure, refers to the amount of energy for essential life (BMR), the energy expended to digest, absorb and convert food, and the energy expended during physical activity.
TWL	total weight loss, can be determined by subtracting pre-

	operative weight from post-operative weight.
UDCA	ursodeoxycholic acid, medication to prevent gallstone formation after bariatric surgery.
VLCD	very low-calorie diet, refers to the diet prior to bariatric surgery in order to shrink the liver. The VLCD is typically around 800-1200 calories a day.

Bariatric terminology

Anastomosis	connection between two tissues in surgical procedures.
Anorexigenic	induction of satiety, for example: leptin is an anorexigenic hormone.
Bariatric	term that refers to different weight loss surgery techniques with the aim to treat obesity.
Comorbidities	diseases that exist in conjunction with obesity.
Dumping	refers to digestive issues when sugar (or fat) enters the small intestine too quickly.
Foamies	refers to the regurgitation of food particles.
Fundus	upper part of the stomach that is removed or bypassed in bariatric surgery procedures.

	This is also the main part where the hunger hormone ghrelin is produced.
Ghrelin	hunger hormone produced in the fundus and small intestine. Ghrelin is often reduced after bariatric surgery leading to a decrease in appetite.
Honeymoon stage	First 12-18 months after bariatric surgery where most excess weight loss is expected.
Intrinsic factor	glycoprotein produced in the stomach that helps to transport and absorb vitamin B12 in the small intestine. Bariatric surgery compromises the production of intrinsic factor (IF), making a vitamin B12 deficiency more likely.
Laparoscopic	type of surgical procedure that allows the surgeon to access the inside of the abdomen without making large incisions in the skin. Also referred to as minimally invasive surgery.
Maintenance stage	from 18 months after bariatric surgery and onwards where the lost weight is expected to be maintained through a new lifestyle.
Neuroplasticity	the ability of the brain to rewire itself.

Orexigenic	induction of hunger, for example: ghrelin is an orexigenic hormone.
Post-op	post-operative, refers to everything after bariatric surgery.
Post-op diet	refers to the post-operative mandatory diet where new foods and textures are slowly re-introduced to allow the pouch's healing and patient recovery.
Pouch	refers to the new small stomach after bariatric surgery.
Pouch reset	refers to the false claim that a liquid diet can "reset" the pouch.
Pouch stretching	referred to as the fear of stretching the pouch after bariatric surgery.
Pre-op	pre-operative, refers to everything before bariatric surgery.
Proffee	a mixture of coffee and a high-protein drink.
Pyloric sphincter	valve between stomach and first part of small intestine to allow a moderate passage of food from the stomach to the small intestine. The pyloric sphincter is absent after mixed procedures like the gastric bypass.

Surgiversary	anniversary of weight loss surgery date.
Surgery twin	somebody who has the same surgery date as you.
Sleeve	refers to the new smaller stomach after the gastric sleeve surgery. The sleeve is shaped like a tube or a "banana".
Transfer addiction	refers to a new-onset addiction that occurs after bariatric surgery when the addiction of food is "transferred" to another substance or activity.

References

Part 1

1. Lowe, M.R., Doshi, S., Katterman, S.N. et al. (2013). Dieting and restrained eating as prospective predictors of weight regain. In: *Frontiers in Psychology*. 2 (4): 577.
2. Schutz, Y., Montain, J., Dulloo, A.G. (2021). Low-carbohydrate ketogenic diets in body weight control: a recurrent plaguing issue of fad diets? In: Obesity Reviews. 22 (S2).
3. Factsheet Metabolic & Bariatric Surgery. The American Society for Metabolic & Bariatric Surgery. Published: 2021.
4. Ivezay, V. Grilo, M. (2018). The complexity of body image following bariatric surgery: a systematic review of the literature. In: *Obesity Reviews*. 19 (8): 1116-1140.
5. Afshar, S., Kelly, S., Seymour, K. et al. (2016). The effects of bariatric procedures on bowel habit. In: *Obesity Surgery*. 26 (10): 2348-2354.
6. Silva Azevado, M., Rodrigues Silva, N. Cunha Mafra, C. et al. (2020). Oral health implications of bariatric surgery in morbidly obese patients: an integrative interview. In: *Obesity Surgery*. 30 (4): 1574-1579.
7. Son, S., Song, J.H., Shin, H., et al. (2022). Prevention of gallstones after bariatric surgery using ursodeoxycholic acid: a narrative in literatures. In: *Journal of Metabolic and Bariatric Surgery*. 11 (2): 30-38.

8. Halawi A, Abiad F, Abbas O. (2013). Bariatric surgery and its effects on the skin and skin diseases. In: *Obesity Surgery*. 23 (3): 408-413.
9. Rojas P, Gosch M, Basfi-fer K, et al. (2011). Alopecia in women with severe and morbid obesity who undergo bariatric surgery. *Nutricion Hospitalaria*. 26 (4): 856-862.
10. Zhang W, Fan, M. et al. (2021). Hair loss after metabolic and bariatric surgery: a systematic review and meta-analyis. In: *Obesity Surgery*. 31 (6): 2649-2659.

Part 2

11. Mechanik J, Apovian C, Brethauer S, et al. (2020). Clinical practical guidelines for the perioperative nutrition, metabolic, and nonsurgical support of patients undergoing bariatric procedures – 2019 update: cosponsored by American association of clinical endocrinologists/American college of endocrinology, the obesity society, American society for metabolic & bariatric Surgery, obesity medicine association, and American society of anesthesiologists. *Surgery for Obesity and Related Diseases*. 16 (2): 175-247.
12. Parrott, M.S., Frank, M.P.H., Rabena, R. et al. (2017). American Society for Metabolic and Bariatric Surgery Integrated Health Nutritional Guidelines for the Surgical Weight Loss Patient 2016 Update: Micronutrients. In: *Surgery for Obesity and Related Diseases*. 13: 727-741.
13. Aillis, L., Blankenship, J. Buffington, C., et al. (2008). ASMBS Bariatric Nutrition Guidelines. In:

Surgery for Obesity and Related Diseases. 4 (5 Suppl): S73-108.

14. Parikh, M., Johnson, J., et al. (2016). ASMBS position statement on alcohol before and after bariatric surgery. In: *Surgery for Obesity and Related Diseases.* 12 (2): 225-230.

15. Vinolas, H., Barnetche, T., Ferrandi, G., et al. (2019). Oral hydration, food intake, and nutritional status before and after bariatric surgery. In: *Obesity Surgery.* 29 (9): 2896-2903.

16. Chaston, T.B., Dixon, J.B. & O'Brien, P.E. (2007). Changes in fat-free mass during significant weight loss: a systematic review. *International Journal of Obesity*: 31(5): 743-750.

17. Canterini C.C., Gaubil-Kaladjian, I., Vatin, S., et al. (2018). Rapid Eating is Linked to Emotional Eating in Obese Women Relieving from Bariatric Surgery. In: *Obesity Surgery*: 28 (2): 526-531.

18. Parkes, E. (2006). Nutritional management of patients after bariatric surgery. *American Journal of the Medical Sciences*: 331 (4); 207-213.

19. Moize V., Andreu A., Rodriguez L., et al. (2013). Protein intake and lean tissue mass retention following bariatric surgery. *Clinical Nutrition.* 32(4): 550-555.

Part 3

20. Chao, A.M., Jastreboff, A.M., White, M.A., et al. (2017). Stress, cortisol and other appetite-related hormones: Prospective prediction of 6-month changes and weight. In: *Obesity.* 25 (4): 713-720.

21. Makris, C.M., Alexandrou, Al, Papatsoutosos, G.E., et al. (2017). Ghrelin and obesity: Identifying gaps and dispelling myths. A reappraisal. In: *In Vivo*. 31 (6): 1047-1050.

22. Terra, X., Auguet, T., Guiu-Jurdao, E., et al. (2013). Long-term changes in leptin, chemerin and ghrelin levels following different bariatric surgery procedures: Roux-en-Y gastric bypass and sleeve gastrectomy. In: *Obesity Surgery*. 23 (11): 1790-1798.

23. Primack, C. (2021). Obesity and sleep. In: *Nursing clinics of North America*. 56 (4): 565-572.

24. Papamargaritis D, Koukoulis G, Sioka E, et al. (2012). Dumping symptoms and incidence of hypoglycaemia after provocation test at 6 and 12 months after laparoscopic sleeve gastrectomy. In: *Obesity Surgery*: 22 (10): 1600-1606.

25. Tzovaras G, Papmargaritis D, Sioka E, et al. (2012). Symptoms suggestive of dumping syndrome after provocation in patients after laparoscopic sleeve gastrectomy. In: *Obesity Surgery*: 22 (1): 23-28.

26. Ukleja, A. (2005). Dumping syndrome: pathophysiology and treatment. In: *Nutrition in Clinical Practice*: 20 (5): 517-525.

27. Friedrich A., Dammus-Machado, A., Meile, T., et al. (2013). Laparoscopic sleeve gastrectomy compared to a multidisciplinary weight loss program for obesity-effects on body composition and protein status. In: *Obesity Surgery*. 23 (12): 1957-1965.

Part 4

28. Pacanowski, C.R., Linde, J.A., & Neumark-Sztainer, D. (2015). Self-weighing: Helpful or harmful for psychological well-being? A review of literature. In: Current Obesity Reports. 4 (1): 65-72.
29. Palascha, A., Kleef van, E. & Trijp van, H.C.M. (2015). How does thinking in black and white terms relate to eating behavior and weight regain? In: *Journal of Health and Psychology*. 20 (5): 638-648.
30. Jong de, J., Vanderschuren L. & Adan, R. (2016). The mesolimbic system and eating addiction: what sugar does and does not do. In: Current Opinion in Behavioral Sciences. 6 (9): 118-216.
31. Making health habitual: the psychology of 'habit formation' and general practice. In: British Journal of General Practice. 62 (605): 664-666.

Part 5

32. Diepenvens, Kl, Haberer, D., Westerterp-Platenga, M. (2008). Different proteins and biopeptides differently affect satiety and anorexigenic/orexigenic hormones in healthy humans. In: *International Journal of Obesity*. 32 (3): 510-518.
33. Guerrero-Hreins, E., Foldi, C.J., Oldfield, B.J. (2022). Gut-brain mechanisms underlying changes in disordered eating behavior after bariatric surgery: a review. In: *Reviews in Endocrine and Metabolic Disorders*. 23 (4): 733-751.

34. Smith, K.E., Orcutt, M. Steffen, K.J. et al. (2019). Loss of control eating and binge eating in the 7 years following bariatric surgery. In: *Obesity Surgery*. 29 (6): 1773-1780.
35. Hao, Z., Mumphrey, M.B., Morisson, C.D. et al. (2016). Does gastric bypass surgery change body weight set point? In: *International Journal of Obesity Supplements*. 6 (1): S37-S43.
36. Voorwinde, V., Steenhuis, I.H.H., Janssen, I.M.C, et al. (2020). Definitions of long-term weight regain and their associations with clinical outcomes. In: *Obesity Surgery*. 30 (20): 527-536.
37. Quercia, I., Dutia, R., Kotler, D.P., et al. (2014). Gastrointestinal changes after bariatric surgery. In: *Diabetes & Metabolism Journal*. 40 (2): 87-94.
38. Athanasiadis, D.I., Kapsampelis, M.A., Monfared, P., et al. (2021). Factors associated with weight regain post-bariatric sugery: a systematic review. In: *Surgical Endoscopy*. 35 (8): 4069-4084.
39. Noria, S.F., Shelby, R.D., Atkins, K.D., et al. (2023). Weight regain after bariatric surgery: scope of the problem, causes, prevention and treatment. In: *Current Diabetes Reports*. 23 (3): 31-42.
40. Grover, B.T., Morell, M.C., Kothari, S.N., et al. (2019). Defining weigh loss after bariatric surgery: a call for standardization. In: *Obesity Surgery*. 29 (11): 3493-3499.

Printed in Great Britain
by Amazon

39476748R00116